Interferon

Interferon

The New Hope for Cancer

Mike Edelhart
with Dr Jean Lindenmann
co-discoverer of Interferon

ORBIS PUBLISHING · LONDON

Interferon

First published in Great Britain in 1982 by
Orbis Publishing Limited, 20-22 Bedfordbury, London WC2

Printed in the United States of America

ISBN: 0-85613-453-8

THIS BOOK IS DEDICATED TO
THE MEMORY OF CAROLE CONTARSY

Acknowledgments

Many people helped put this book together. Leslie Miner and Robin Webster helped enormously with their reporting from England. Diana Bingham slaved over a complex manuscript and a heap of difficult interview tapes. Adele Paroni of the American Cancer Society was extremely cooperative as was Joan Chin at M.D. Anderson Hospital.

My particular thanks go to all the scientists who gave of their time to talk with us about interferon. They were the key to getting the fullest possible view of this complex situation.

And most of all, my thanks to Jean Lindenmann, without whom, in every sense, this book never would have existed.

Preface

Mike Edelhart's valiant attempt at a balanced description of a fast-moving scientific adventure succeeds without unduly fanning too many expectations or quenching too many hopes. It manages to present a vivid account of the present state of knowledge and ignorance in a field which has become distorted by gratuitous speculations and by equally unfounded misgivings.

Inevitably, such a non-technical report leaves the impression that the exciting stages of scientific research are those that eventually emerge into the limelight of public attention. This of course is not true. If some people feel attracted to research, it is because its real excitements lie precisely in those phases of groping exploration that must seem tedious and dull to an outside observer. A few vainglorious moments of triumph fade fast; the satisfaction of an intellectually honest effort is more enduring. But it is perhaps just as well that this aspect of scientific work hardly ever comes through in popular writing. There ought to be secret joys that science reserves exclusively to those bold enough or naive enough to answer its call.

While reading this book, and particularly the chapter that deals with my own contribution, I was reminded of a passage by the former grand old lady of French letters, Colette: "Is it always so? This half-success, this half-catastrophe?" Indeed, how could human endeavors lead to anything but tainted achievements? I will settle for half a success, and even for much less, any time, provided the catastrophes remain within bounds.

JEAN LINDENMANN

Zurich
January 1981

CONTENTS

The Agony of Expectations

On March 25, 1980 a small parcel arrived in Glasgow, Scotland on a routine, commercial flight from Denmark. It looked like nothing so much as a small wrapped trinket, a souvenir for the folks back home. Yet it was rushed from the plane with a tight-lipped haste, spun past customs and hurtled through the narrow, gray streets of the dour Scottish town.

Interferon. A minuscule amount, enough to treat two small boys for an insignificant length of time. The tiny vials in the package had cost almost $3,000. Their destination was the august hospital, Victoria Infirmary.

Dr. Tom McAllister, of Glasgow's Royal Hospital for Sick Children, had spent months begging Dr. Kierulfe Neilson, head of Denmark's interferon laboratory, to spare him a measly portion of the precious, rare substance. He had two young patients completely beyond help. Their cancers would certainly snuff their lives, after first exacting a vicious toll of pain and disfigurement. McAllister felt he had to try something. He turned to interferon.

When the drug arrived McAllister said: "The merciful action of the Danes confirms that doctors are holding on to the finest principles and putting the suffering of ordinary humanity before money. I had feared this would become a rich man's drug. The Shah (of Iran) is willing to pay anything. But I'm so grateful Britain's first patient will be an ordinary boy who desperately needs the drug as his chance to stay alive."

He began treatments immediately, and on April 12, 1980, McAllister held a press conference that rocked Britain's medical establishment. One of his patients, a victim of inner-ear cancer so severe it had completely obscured his face, "was able to see out of his left eye for the first time in two months and his left ear became more noticeable. The change in his general state of health has been enormous. He is a new boy altogether."

The English press went crazy. Cancer cured! Magic drug saves boy! Interferon works wonders! Miracle in Scotland!

And the phones in Glasgow hospitals and the hushed halls of the Imperial Cancer Research Fund rang off their hooks. Frantic family members pleaded for interferon to save their loved ones. Victims wept and offered anything they owned—everything—for a drop of the miracle drug. Angry seekers stormed medical halls convinced the testers were hoarding it all for themselves.[1]

Inundated, Glasgow's Health Board begged cancer sufferers to stop calling. Stunned, the biological research community fought back, diffidently at first and then firmly.

"I think it was used in treatment far too early," said Professor Kenneth Calman of Glasgow University's oncology department. "We don't even know what dosage to give. These questions must all be answered before using the drug for treatment."

"What must be realized," ventured Dr. Nigel Kemp, scientific secretary of the Cancer Research Campaign, "is that there is not a lot of interferon about at the moment, and we feel that what there is should be used in clinically controlled trials."

The definitive pronouncement came from the Coordinating Committee on Cancer Research, the overlord of Britain's research effort. It was sympathetic, but firm:

"Because cancer is so common—some 145,000 die of it each year in the United Kingdom—few can be unaware, from personal experience, of the intense distress of the families and friends of cancer sufferers. There must therefore be every sympathy with the feelings of those who have taken hope from press, radio and television reports and who have made desperate efforts to obtain supplies of interferon. Nonetheless, we must emphasize that, because there is so little interferon available—and that at a very high cost—the first priority must be to use it in carefully designed clinical trials to establish how effective it is, while at the same time pressing on with research to find better ways to make it."

The scientific counterattack dampened the fire only slightly. More daunting was news that McAllister's first patient had died after just two weeks of treatment. And "Daniel," the boy whose cancer had seemed so remarkably improved, died in mid-July.

"All I can say," stated McAllister, "is that we tried out best."

What is the substance that can inflame such passions and engender such hopes? It is a sinuous, sticky protein found in most higher animals and virtually all human cells. It is produced only rarely in the body and then in such minute quantities that detecting its presence requires enormous effort in the lab. And it is so rare outside of the body that a pound of purified interferon was once estimated to be worth $20 billion. Blood from 270 donors is needed to produce enough interferon to treat one person for a few weeks. It has been known for twenty-four years, but has been so hard to come by during that time that only a skeleton crew of dedicated researchers kept it alive in science at all.

But today this small-time protein is thought to have startling capabilities against viruses, including the common cold, and greater potential as a cancer treatment than anything to come on the scene in the last ten years. It could revolutionize cancer therapy—if we could only get our hands on a substantial amount for testing.

The soaring hopes for interferon are counterbalanced by the intense frustration rising from its rarity in the face of cancer's steady spread. While other major causes of death are being reduced by science, cancer marches on, killing more people each year. Four hundred thousand Americans die of cancer annually, and one million are diagnosed as having it. That means that one out of four American families has been touched by the scourge. They have seen mothers, fathers, aunts, uncles, or siblings succumb slowly to their own rampaging systems. Even more distressing are the disfiguring, debilitating effects of the supposedly humane treatments for the condition. A relative's hair turns shockingly white almost overnight, then falls out. He loses interest in life. He's always tired, and is often nauseous and depressed. And doctors point to statistics saying, "see, we're faring better against cancer now." But the families don't think their cancer-ridden relative is really living, and they don't think the doctors can really help. "They didn't let him die," said one relative of a cancer victim, "but they couldn't keep him alive."

Interferon, in use so far, is keeping people alive. Experiments have shown it effective at shrinking tumors and stopping their spread—without the terrible side-effects that cause people to dread chemotherapy and radiation even more than cancer itself.

When any such medication appears on the scene with even the

smallest hint of effectiveness against cancer, people want to try it in lieu of the damaging, existing therapies, or after the accepted treatments have failed. They don't care if the treatment is experimental; the non-experimental treatments do such damage that something untried doesn't seem too risky by comparison. And if it doesn't work, it certainly can't worsen a situation already terminal.

But interferon, whatever its abilities, is virtually unattainable. Right now the number of cancer patients who receive it is so small they register as only the smallest percentage point of the world's victims. In fact, there isn't enough interferon now on the entire planet to treat all the cancer victims in a single city.

When the public bellows, "try it, no matter what the cost," scientists must holler back, "we can't." People feel cheated. They wonder about conspiracies to withhold effective treatments that would cut down on the brisk medical business of treating cancer cases. They rage against the impotence of science. In bars and country clubs the question is asked, "if we can send men to the moon, why can't we find a cure for cancer?" The question grows from frightened desperation, with experience often gained spookily close at hand.

In this charged atmosphere, the public awaits the appearance of the breakthrough that will make the problem go away. We have been conditioned to expect it. Enter interferon in a flash of big money research funds and apparently unheard-of capabilities. The reaction is almost inescapable. It's like a run on a bank. Once the process has begun, no rational explanation will do. The public, needing to believe in a cure for cancer, chose to believe in interferon and to create incredible pressure on scientists to support them. "You know it works," they cried, "use it! Save us and our families!"

During all this din, researchers are trying diligently to determine just what interferon can and cannot do, how it works, what its true worth is. They struggle to stick to the long-standing, formal procedures for evaluating a new medical treatment, under the added burden of a minuscule supply for testing. They walk the thin line between being too pessimistic—which will cut funding—and too optimistic—which will further inflame public impatience at not being able to get it.

And, most painfully, they are forced to play God. Researchers must select from the clamoring multitude of cancer victims the very, very few who will receive interferon experimentally. In the case of any hopeful medication this choice is hard; with interferon it is infinitely harder.

This is true partially because hopes for interferon are so much higher than they have ever been for a potential cancer drug. The positive publicity and rumors have actually convinced many people—including many cancer patients—that the end to their anxieties is at hand. As much as scientists caution that interferon recipients are taking a gamble, a vast group imagines that those chosen for tests are actually receiving a cure.

In addition, since the supply of interferon is so minute—enough to treat, at most, a thousand or so people in the entire world—the number of patients accepted for testing is far fewer than researchers would ordinarily recommend. The number of possible recipients is so small it verges on the statistically meaningless.

As one cancer researcher put it: "For all practical purposes, interferon as a medical treatment does not exist. It is not a potential choice for a cancer patient today. They have as much chance of being hit by lightning as receiving interferon right now."

The ethical pressure on interferon researchers is enormous. The choices they make are unfair to far more people than they are beneficial. Whoever they accept will be overly elated and whoever they reject will be deeply depressed without just cause. The patient is squeezed between interferon's hopeful, expansive future and its limited, tentative present.

The greatest pain falls, of course, upon the cancer victims, their families, and the researchers who have to explain, quietly and logically, why the cancer can't be treated with a drug they are convinced could help, or even cure them.

As the journal *Nature* asked: "How does one set about telling a patient suffering from cancer that there may at some stage be a more effective treatment than at present, but that it cannot be generally available for some years, by which time he or she may be dead?"[2]

Virtually every serious cancer victim wants to know about getting interferon today. "We tried to put a lid on the hysteria that has been generated about interferon," states Dr. Charles G. Moertel of the Mayo Clinic in Rochester, Minnesota. "We seldom see a cancer patient without being asked about interferon treatment."

At the American Cancer Society, Dr. Frank Rauscher, the director of research, says, "Here at my office I receive at least seventy phone calls each week from patients, their parents and so forth. It's very difficult, of course, it's just heartrending as a matter of fact that all we can say is that it's a research program and we need to have more information and more interferon, for that matter, before we can even consider the ethics of recommending it to individual patients.

"The unquenchable desire for interferon by cancer victims," Rauscher states, "is my continuing nightmare."

"We're being absolutely bombarded," says Dr. Eliott Osserman of Columbia University's interferon testing program. "It's one of the most frustrating experiences of my whole medical career. You want to do good, to help people, and there's nothing you can do."

Dr. Jordan Gutterman, of Houston's M.D. Anderson Hospital, was forced to get an unlisted phone number because of all the interferon-seeking calls. "Whenever a cancer patient or his family reads an article, they call in. People will auction their homes, do anything to get some of the stuff. It can be harassing at times."

At the Memorial Sloan-Kettering Cancer Center, Dr. Susan Krown is beseiged by interferon-hungry cancer victims. "People have read things that make them think this is some kind of miracle cure," she says. "Because interferon is scarce and our studies are limited, we have to turn down patients every day who have invested a lot of emotional energy in trying to get interferon. When they can't get it they feel like they're being cheated out of something that's the answer for them. It's sad."

Nor do the entreaties come just from simple folk. Both Rauscher and Mathilde Krim, director of Sloan-Kettering's interferon lab, have been pressured by U.S. Senators, Congressmen and influential business leaders trying to get interferon for themselves or relatives. "It is touchy," says Dr. Krim, "when you have to say no to someone who controls your purse strings."

In England, the situation is much the same. "People involved clinically have found it very disconcerting to be approached, often in very distressing circumstances, by people who feel that here's something that can help them. They have to say, 'no, it can't yet.' And you hear some quite, quite awful stories about the lengths people will go to because they think it might be the answer for them," states Dr. Walter Bodmer, chief of Britain's Imperial Cancer Research Fund.

English researchers had the particularly painful task of coping with the outpouring of response to the wildly ballyhooed Glasgow incident. It has left many British researchers, even those with supreme confidence in interferon, shaken and bitter.

"I think this Glasgow case is absolutely disgraceful," Bodmer glowers. "When you see a front-page article on two cases in Glasgow, where there have been lots of other cases that have been done under at least reasonably controlled conditions it makes you angry. And then to hear that interferon is hopeless because those patients died at the same time as you're coping with entreaties from patients who demand the treatment is infuriating."

Dr. Derek C. Burke of Warwicke University, who is one of the earliest interferon researchers, states strongly that "this (experiment) was an immoral thing to do. I'm not saying his information was spurious. I think it's quite likely there was a transitory effect of interferon. But it's hopeless to try and save somebody like that, just hopeless. And raising expectations that way just tears people apart and makes it difficult for us to reasonably study and report findings.

"If ill-conceived experiments like this fail, they can take the serious work of the field with them. The backlash can finish the field and we might lose something that will be of value. So what we've got to try to do is be reasonable."

As a result of Glasgow, Burke states, "We get a lot of letters from victims. I had one yesterday: A wife terminally ill, in a chair, unable to walk, cancer all through the bone and in the back. Young couple. And can I help? Please? I can't. None of us can. All we can do is work it around but there's no way we can help any."

A few doctors, like Dr. McAllister in Glasgow, have given in to the blandishments and use interferon as a treatment. Most scientists, though, have held firm. But they don't like the situation. They worry that the public clamor over the drug will make it impossible to conduct adequate research to find out just what interferon can do. They fear the public's disinclination to wait for full scientific information will result in a fierce backlash that could dry up funding and stop work of real importance.

Scientists have a strange approach-avoidance conflict with public acclaim and informational hunger. When interferon appears on the covers of *Time* and *Life*, they don't know whether they should be proud or bolt the door and take the phone off the hook. The dissonance is annoying.

"Media interest has helped bring interferon to the public's attention, but it has also brought the danger of rising expectations," stated Dr. Jordan Gutterman, one of the field's "big guns." "Many people don't realize that this substance is still extremely experimental, and not available for widespread use. I think that interferon has probably received more publicity than it deserves at this stage of the game."

This distressing dilemma was played out in an editorial in *Nature* entitled, "What Not to Say About Interferon":

"The physicians are not concerned to shuffle off their professional responsibilities; rather, they are anxious to protect the patients and their relatives from such needless distress as there is bound to be when it is believed that a potentially beneficial drug is being withheld. It is no comfort to those concerned to know that the quantities of interferon now available are sufficient only to sustain a handful of clinical trials here and there . . . it can take very little ingenuity for the general public to discover that many professional people are indeed excited about interferon because of the possibility that it may have a role to play in the treatment of at least some kinds of cancer. . . . The questions for the professional community, physicians included, is therefore not that of avoiding publicity, but of making sure that the harmful consequences of publicity are avoided."[3]

Maintaining this standard presents doctors and scientists with a taxing challenge. And most in the interferon field have made serious attempts to meet it. The result has been statements that are either cautious or equivocating, depending upon your point of view. They have also been open to interpretation, thus fanning the flames they were supposed to still.

"So far the experimental use of interferon as an anti-cancer agent for specific kinds of cancer is more or less a shot in the dark. When these experimental decisions are made, one asks whether there is an alternative treatment; if so, patients must always receive the best available therapy. In the case of (certain cancers) there was no proven, or very promising treatment available and it was felt that interferon might, therefore, be beneficial to these patients. And so the question of whether or not to use interferon experimentally is a complex of practical and theoretical considerations," according to Dr. Robert M. Friedman of the National Institutes of Health.

"We don't know how effective interferon is going to prove to be," concurs Dr. Frank Rauscher of the American Cancer Society. "We don't know the proper regimen to improve effectiveness. We don't know how long the therapeutic effect is going to last. It's important for people to realize that this is a *research* program.

"The only way to determine which diseases are the most responsive is through clinical trials. And it is also only through clinical trials that we can determine—for any specific disease—the most suitable type of interferon, the optimal dosage, the most effective route of administration and the appropriate duration of treatment. It is possible that interferon alone will not provide the kind of dramatic breakthrough in clinical medicine that was made, for example, by penicillin."

Still, the fact remains that in various parts of the world there are several dozen people who are alive today most likely through beneficial responses to interferon. On a statistical scale, a few dozen individuals means nothing. But on the scale of hope it means quite a lot.

Interferon helped these people beat the grim odds against them. They are among the tiny band who have been given the chance to receive the drug. If more people could get it, how many more could beat the odds against them?

It is a question that has not been answered, and won't be until late 1981 at the earliest, when interferon produced through genetic engineering will explode onto the research scene expanding testing incredibly. But it cries out for answering *now* and a public fearful of the spectre of cancer waits with barely restrained impatience for a definitive word.

While the ultimate answer will take time to achieve, more limited questions can be dealt with now. What does science really know about interferon? How well has the drug worked against cancer and a host of other serious diseases, including the common cold and rabies? Why did it take twenty-three years for science to "discover" a substance of such unmatched potential power? Exactly what is happening with interferon today?

By answering these specific questions, we can sketch in the outlines of the broader speculation: What will this strange new drug mean to me and my family?

PART ONE

WHAT IT IS, HOW IT WORKS

chapter 1

THE FIRST LINE OF DEFENSE

1

Interferon is a protein our bodies produce regularly. Its function: to protect our cells from the ravages of invasion. When cells in the body are threatened by a virus, or by the challenges of cancer tumors, they turn into highly efficient interferon production factories in a last-ditch effort to save as many surrounding cells as possible.

Interferon is the body's picket line, the first line of defense against a concentrated assault. It can't (and isn't designed to) hold off attackers forever. But it fends them off while greater forces muster for the most effective counterattack.

Understanding all of interferon's abilities, including those against cancer cells, rests on comprehending how the protein gallops into action when viruses attack. Somehow, though no one is certain just how, interferon's anti-viral actions are linked intrinsically to its potency against tumors.

The wonder of the power that freezes viruses in place and shrinks some tumors can best be seen by viewing a genetic invasion from a cell's point of view. To the individual, a virus attack is usually just a nuisance. But to the cells involved, it entails, almost literally, pillage and slavery leading to a horrible death.

Viruses do not merely invade human cells; they force them to exert themselves to death in the production of new virus material. The complex chain of rogue genetic materials that comprise a virus first attaches itself to the victim-cell's wall. It rips away the cell's protective layers and burrows into the heart of the host. There, the domineering invader shoots out sharp genetic orders to the cell's nucleus. The ordinary operations of cellular life are suspended; the occupier's orders supercede the normal genetic code.

The infected cell begins slapping together material for new versions of the controlling virus. Completely overpowered, it gives no precedence to its own nutritional needs or bodily function. Instead, the cell is riveted to the production of self-made viruses. Unable to stop its forced labor, the cell swells, its walls strain, bulge, and finally erupt, releasing a horde of viruses into intercellular fluid to beset surrounding cells. The viruses surge onward, infecting yet more cells, leaving behind the spent, dead remnants of the plundered victim cells.

It would seem that this process would expand throughout the body, inexorably turning the entire system into a gigantic virus production factory and killing the host organism. But it doesn't happen. Viruses, by and large, are self-limiting; they eventually succumb to the body's defenses. And they can't gang up on the system; only one virus strain at a time can make its play for bodily domination.

The reason for this is the intricate silent alarm system nature has programmed into the genetic material of virtually every cell. It assures that the virus-infected cell does not die in vain. This is the interferon system, in which dying cells broadcast desperate warnings to those around them of the invasion and induce them to protect themselves against intrusion.

HOW INTERFERON WORKS

In a home burglar alarm system, an electric current energizes a magnet that keeps the lights from flashing and the bells from clanging. When a burglar opens the door, he breaks the current, cancelling the magnet and releasing the cacophony of alarms. The cell's interferon system works in much the same way.

All cells, researchers have determined, have locked into their genetic codes two conflicting orders. In humans, chromosome 5 or 9, of our twenty-three pairs of cell-controlling strands, contains the genetic statement that leads to production of interferon. Elsewhere among the chromosomes lies a countermanding order that blocks initiation of the interferon imperative.

During the ordinary operation of the cell the two orders hold each other in check and the cell produces no interferon. Under certain circumstances, however, the "halt" order is stripped away, the existing "produce" order snaps into action, and interferon results.

The chromosomes don't actually manufacture interferon. Rather, the genetic "produce" order brings about formation of a long strand of a nucleic acid called messenger-RNA. The name derives from the fact that this chemical chain works as a blueprint for the formation of proteins. It attracts different chemicals to link together in a specific order. When the linking is through, a protein has been formed.

The interferon protein is a relatively long one, larger than insulin and other common members of the clan. The details of its makeup are not well known. But generally interferon seems to resemble other proteins in every way—except its effects. The impact of most proteins is quite specific; they work in a tightly defined area of the cell's life. But interferon protein is capable of completely transforming the cell; its potency reaches into *every crevice* of cellular existence.

This uniquely broad range of power is the key to interferon's importance. It is a common, naturally occurring substance with the ability to control the cells that produce it. Not one part of the cell, but the entire unit. Not one kind of cell, but virtually every cell.

Interferon is the first strong, tangible evidence that our cells create chemicals of universal efficacy. Interferon's mode of operation holds promise for shifting medical thinking about cures away from external controls and toward internal modulators of cells and systems.

TYPES OF INTERFERON

For the sake of simplicity, interferon will be referred to as a single substance. Keep in mind, however, that there is no one such substance. Interferon is a name that covers several different proteins of different structures, strengths, and capabilities. Their common factor is that they control cells in the face of viral invasion.

Leukocyte interferon is the most common today. Leukocytes are white blood cells, from which this protein is derived. Early interferon experiments were almost entirely concerned with leukocyte material because that was the only known source for human interferon.

More is known about leukocyte interferon than other types because it has been used so much more. Some research today indicates that this substance (also called alpha interferon) is actually composed of as many as sixteen different proteins linked or twined together. Most interferon produced until very recently came in the form of a chemical soup that was mostly junk with the tiniest hint of interferon in it. As scientists have studied and purified this soup they have seen increasing evidence that the interferon effect may be altered by the balance of other proteins in the chemical mix along with the single strand that is classically "interferon."

This may mean that other elements besides the protein will be required for a strong effect. It might also mean that shifts in surrounding proteins might alter the effects from a single type of interferon. "It may turn out to be like having pears and oranges," says Dr. Norman Finter of Britain's Burroughs-Wellcome Research Labs. "Both are fruit, but you need their separate attributes mixed together to make a fruit salad."

Fibroblast interferon (also called beta interferon) comes from connective tissues in our muscles. It turned up in experiments performed in 1965, acting as interferon in virus handling abilities, but reacting differently than the leukocyte protein in many basic lab tests. Fibroblast interferon comes from very placid, stable cells. Such a stable source makes it reasonable that muscle tissue interferon would make an eminently safe form of treatment. It also offers some production advantages, since chemicals have been found that induce interferon in fibroblasts but not leukocytes.

There are indications that the differences in interferons are more than structural. It appears that interferons may be most effective against cells similar to the ones that made them. Fibroblast interferon, for example, seems to work best against tumors in skin and muscle tissues, while leukocyte interferon has had somewhat better luck against blood and bone marrow diseases. It seems there is something coded into the structure of each type that focuses its activity better in certain types of cells.

Researchers looking for an easier, cheaper way to make interferon by using cell cultures, found that a laboratory cell line called Namalva created an interferon called *lymphoblastoid* that acted pretty much like leukocyte interferon. There might have been more wild exuberance about this finding if Namalva wasn't a research cell strain descended from an unfortunate African boy who had suffered from Burkitt's lymphoma, a cancer of the lymph nodes.

Incredible as it sounds, this interferon was produced by cancer cells—or more accurately, cells from a cancer victim which had been kept alive in the laboratory. Scientists routinely maintain the cells of several long dead cancer victims in laboratories for use in cancer cell and other experiments. Cancer cells are eternal; unlike regular cells they will multiply and prosper in cell culture medium forever, which means researchers never have to go out and fetch a new supply. The ones that have traditionally responded most evenly and accurately to testing are kept around labs like any other standard testing substance.

The Namalva cells used to produce lymphoblastoid interferon are descended from cancerous lymph cells that had degraded to their undifferentiated state. Researchers in England were intrigued by the cells because the eternally reproducing cancer connection meant they could manufacture lymphoblastoid protein far faster than any other kind of interferon. But the worry about using cells descended from a cancer as the production medium for a cancer treatment worried other scientists.

Norman Finter, director of the lymphoblastoid program at Britain's Burroughs-Wellcome labs sees no reason for concern about lymphoblastoid interferon. "There's no actual certainty these are tumor cells. They came from a child with a tumor, but that's semantics. In any case, you treat them as though they were tumor cells; you double over backward to prove safety and provide purity. I think we've convinced the authorities in this country and I think we'll do so in other countries. We've proven that our process of purification eliminates viruses, cancer cells, everything to be worried about."

Even so, lymphoblastoid interferon is not yet approved for use in the United States. Even at far less cost, an interferon produced from malignant cells would have problems getting accepted as a research tool or medication in the United States. Unless official attitudes change, these drawbacks could outweigh any advantages.

The most mysterious and ultimately, perhaps, the most important interferons are those created by the lymphocytes, the stalwart cells of the immune system. Called *immune interferon* or T-interferon (for the thymus gland which controls lymphocytes), these proteins arise in the face of challenges to the immune system. Despite their poorly understood link with cancer regulating systems, these interferons may be crucial in combatting tumors. For the moment, though, they remain as much an object of speculation as of verified fact.

The apparent differences in all the interferons may turn out, in time, to be the result of structural variables that have nothing to do with any anti-viral or -tumor response. Many experts now believe that the interferon molecules all bear a lot of dead weight, that the actual work is handled by a compact core of amino acids common to all the different kinds of interferon. It has already been shown that the sugars at either end of interferons are not involved in the protective mechanism; similarly, much of the rest of the long molecule is residue of the organic processes that made it. The necessary section for viral protection and tumor reduction may be a mere fraction of the whole.

This means, of course, that stripping away the extraneous material could produce a pure interferon, which we will call *minimal interferon*, with maximum impact and minimum drawbacks. Minimal interferon could eliminate one of the drug's greatest limitations throughout its history—species specificity. This means that only human interferon can be used to treat humans. While most virus treatments are produced by culturing an antibody and then growing it in animals or eggs, then purifying what you've grown and diluting it to the proper dosage for treatment, interferon can't be handled in this way, much the pity.

Early interferon researchers found, to their chagrin, that mouse interferon worked only in mice, rabbit interferon only in rabbits, and human interferon only in humans. It appeared impossible to use animals as a growing medium for human interferon; you needed human cells, a rare and expensive commodity in a human-centered world.

Recent research has found, however, that interferon is not entirely species specific, but the effectiveness is strongest in the home species and quite unpredictable outside of it.

The notion of an interferon core, however, raises the possibility that cross-species limitation is a result of the extraneous interferon material and might have nothing to do with the core. The active part of interferon might be the same for all animals—plants, too—and a properly stripped molecule would work in any creature, no matter where it had been cultivated. . . .

WAYS INTERFERON PROTECTS THE BODY

Just how does interferon stimulate the body's defenses against virus diseases and cancer tumors? With a single basic capability: Interferon warns cells of a genetic invader in their midst and warns the body about activities in the hearts of cells that could damage it.

Interferon attacks nothing and kills nothing. It does not have much effect on the cell that produces it. The protein's powers are for the benefit of surrounding cells. It is a sentry whose warnings make the community better able to defend itself.

When a virus attacks a cell, it injects rogue, viral-RNA into the cell fluid. Most often, this alien strand contains a double loop of RNA, as compared to the healthy cell's single stranded messengers. This twist of genetic material contains the virus' instructions to the invaded cell. They will halt normal cell functions and lead to the fevered, eventually fatal, production of more virus.

But the viral-RNA somehow sets off the "interferon-production" message on the chromosomes. Through a complicated process of protein and enzyme links that is not yet fully understood, something in the virus messenger strips away the long standing "hold" on interferon creation.

As it is being subjugated by the virus, the cell's interferon order causes production of a messenger-RNA molecule for interferon. The long chain of chemicals joined together by this messenger-RNA forms the core of interferon, the protein part of the molecule, which is called *interferoid*.

The interferoid is transported, like a spy behind enemy lines, through the cellular fluid, toward the cell wall. There, sugar molecules are added to both ends in a process called glycolization. The glycolized molecule is interferon. It is squirted into the intercellular fluid and heads out to warn other cells of the viral invasion.

Dr. Mathilde Krim of Sloan-Kettering has called interferon "a kind of chemical Paul Revere," which is a surprisingly accurate description. Like the night-riding silversmith, interferon has no power to stop the approaching invasion—no chemical guns or soldiers. It is merely a message carrier and initiator of the body's defense.

Once the interferon messenger is loose among the cells, it searches for a surface receptor that it can bind to. Surface receptors are genetically coded chemicals on the cell walls, apparently engineered by chromosome 21 in humans, that bind with interferon and lock it in position to transmit its vital message.

Evidence indicates that interferon, unlike a virus, doesn't need to get inside a cell to transmit its message. Instead, it stimulates from without the production of special anti-viral proteins within the cell. Somehow, interferon induces a chromosome in the cell to create a messenger-RNA that puts together the invasion-fighting chemical.

This chemical, keep in mind, is *not* interferon. It is an entirely different protein produced by the genetic controls inside a cell that interferon binds to. The anti-viral protein also doesn't protect the cell

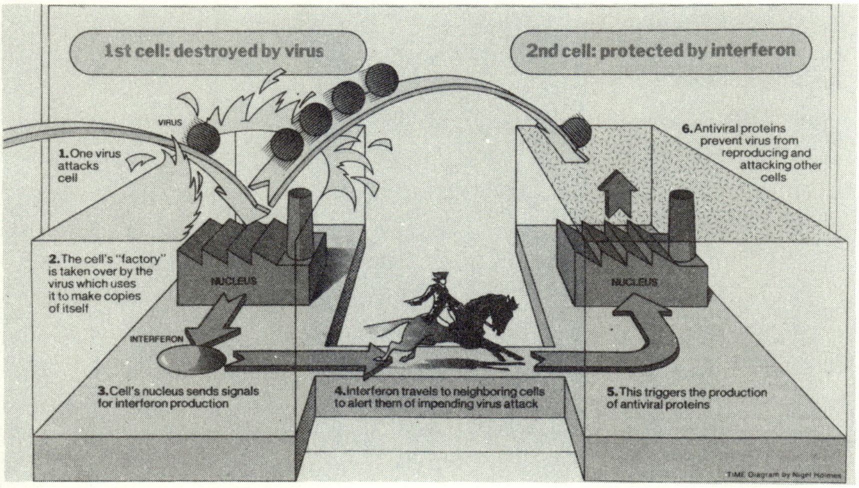

Diagram from *Time* magazine by Nigel Holmes.

against the initial inroads of a virus. The nefarious strain will still bind to the cell wall and inject itself into the cell material. But once there, it will be stymied. The interferon-warned cell will not respond to the virus' genetic demands. Alone, surrounded by the cell's defense forces, the virus will die, its mission unfulfilled.

Stonewalling viral replication in cells isn't interferon's only response, either. The protective protein creates a number of secondary reactions to keep cells functioning even though under attack. It slows the rate of cell multiplication, thus impeding viral spread through the body. Lowered cell division rates carry important ramifications for interferon's anti-tumor effects as well. Interferon also produces significant changes in the structure of a cell's surface and sustenance systems that appear to increase the chances for survival against any type of altering situation.

Another interferon effect, and one that opens up the wide realm of the protein's anti-cancer possibilities, centers on the immune system. Immunology, the study of the body's ability to rid itself of invaders, is a science still in swaddling. Only with the most recent advances in genetic understanding and cellular study has any picture emerged of this microscopic, incredibly complex system. Even now, understanding of immune responses is filled with yawning gaps in knowledge.

So, the details of where interferon fits in this picture are virtually non-existent. But the broader outlines of startling effects have been seen. For instance, it is known that when interferon is given early in an immune response, it lowers the body's ability to reject the interloper; given late in the cycle, however, interferon increases the immune response. This is an interesting paradox which, right now, defies complete explanation.

The interferon-immune connection is deeply fascinating to researchers because the spread of cancer cells seems to be linked somehow to a suppression of the body's natural ability to fight off unnatural elements—its ability to make itself immune to invasion. Interferon has been shown to react against tumors in mice, apparently by heightening the body's own natural defenses against such cells.

Here again, interferon's role seems to be as coach rather than player. Interferon doesn't attack tumor cells. It doesn't shrink tumors. It doesn't, as noted above, always increase immune response. When interferon is put directly into contact with tumor cells outside of the body, little or nothing happens. In the body, however, interferon creates significant anti-tumor effects, at least in experiments using mice.

An indirect influence is at work here. Rather than attacking the tumor cells itself, interferon is stimulating the body to do something of its own to eliminate them. A notion of how the body uses interferon against tumors has arisen only in the past couple of years with the discovery of a strange bodily enforcer called the NK—the *natural killer cell.*

NK cells aren't the body's only killers of invasive forces. Macrophages, giant white blood cells, surround and gobble certain unwanted elements in the blood. And killer cells (as opposed to natural killer cells) attack and demolish invading cells when they have been activated by specific antibodies—antibodies that make it possible for killer cells to recognize their targets.

NK cells, however, require no antibody to get them started. How they work is not yet understood, but what they do is pretty clear. NK cells float through the body on constant alert against abnormal cells. Like a SWAT team, they rush in with "high firepower" when a situation is on the verge of getting out of hand.

The importance of these roving avengers against tumors was first discovered in studies of mice with deficient immune systems, so-called nude mice. Nude mice, it was surmised, should have higher rates of cancer than other mice because their weak immune systems would collapse sooner under the burden of early tumors. To researchers' surprise, this turned out to be quite false. The reason appears to be that nude mice have normal numbers of natural killer cells. Somehow the NK cells hold down tumor occurrence even when the rest of the immune system is deficient.

When interferon is present in the body, NK cell activity leaps; this is in contrast to other killer cells where levels stay about the same. This, experts suspect, begins to explain how interferon marshalls the body's defenses against a tumor, and also provides a second method by which the protective protein wipes out viruses.

The presence of interferon in the neighborhood of a tumor is believed to work like a beacon on a foggy night. The patrolling NK cells pick up the distress call and move toward the area. Meanwhile, the interferon is exercising its cell-division-slowdown capabilities to hold down growth of the invader as much as possible until help arrives. The NK cells actually eradicate the tumor cells, though how this is done remains quite hazy.

The NK-interferon partnership strikes down viruses in a similar manner. Virus-infected cells are recognized as alien cells by the body. When interferon floods an area infected by virus, it not only produces all the cellular changes already mentioned, but also calls in the NK cells for a massive "mop-up" of virus-infected cells.

For all its potency, interferon has little staying power in the body. As soon as interferon production begins, a regulatory clock begins ticking. And after a few hours, new orders blocking interferon transcription and breaking up messenger-RNA take hold. From a fast peak, interferon fades steadily away and is gone entirely the day after it was induced.

On the one hand, this worries interferon researchers because it raises the possibility that long-term treatment with interferon could generate dangerous side effects. The body may be protecting itself from these developments by wiping interferon out of the system quickly. Under some circumstances, the fading interferon pattern has been found actually to help in treatment. If some cells are given a small dose of interferon, and then challenged with a second larger dose at the proper time (after the first has begun to fade), the cells put out a startling spurt of interferon by themselves. This is called *super-induction;* its value lies in the fact that it raises the chance to extend limited interferon supplies by letting the body make up some of the dosage itself.

If interferon can modulate the growth of cancer tumors, why doesn't it nip cancer in the bud? It probably does, says Dr. Derek Burke of Warwicke University. "You can easily say that interferon does work against cancer colonies in the body and we only see the cases where it doesn't work. We know that you need multiple events in order to initiate a tumor. Each of the events is intrinsically rather unlikely. You need the whole sequence of rather rare events to produce a tumor. This is why cancer takes so long to develop, why cancer tends to be a disease of old age. All of this suggests that there is a mechanism for blocking these rather rare events and that the mechanism gets less efficient as we get older.

"So, maybe interferon is working and what we see in tumor growth is the breakdown in some rather subtle link in the immune system which is normally modulated by interferon."

Dr. Norman Finter of Britain's Burroughs-Wellcome labs believes that cancers manage to sneak past the interferon control system. "It's an insidious change in the natural cell that the body doesn't recognize. The change from a normal cell to a cancer cell is a slight mutation. Then there's another mutation and another and then the body picks it up because it has become sufficiently different, but it's already too late to control without outside help. It has escaped the system that stimulates production of interferon until it establishes itself."

Just how interferon manages to block virus and cancer genetic messages inside a cell has been a matter of much scientific head scratching. It was believed that the protein had to block either the invader's messenger-RNA or the proteins the RNA encoded. But which?

Recently, Dr. Charles E. Samuel of the University of California at Santa Barbara reported that, at least in some cases, the block comes between the RNA and its proteins. He stated that two enzymes generated by the presence of interferon make it impossible for the RNA to go through the necessary steps to create a protein, and then tear it up. The first enzyme, called *protein kinase*, jumps ahead of the RNA and tinkers with a chemical that forms one of the first links in the translation chain. In its altered form the chemical can no longer bind with the RNA, and so protein creation is stymied. At the same time, interferon initiates a process that produces a stringy molecule with the tongue twister name oligoadenylic acid. This is a nucleic acid made up entirely of adenine, one of the basic building blocks of our genes. The presence of this adenine chain activates creation of an enzyme that tears up messenger-RNA. Such enzymes are called ribonucleases. The ribonuclease attacks the messenger-RNA and breaks it down before any proteins can be manufactured. The result: a frustrated, dead virus.

A fascinating offshoot of Samuel's scenario is his answer to the question: Why do the enzymes wreck only viral-RNA and not all the RNA in the cell? Of course, if the enzymes did attack RNA indiscriminantly, the cure for the virus would be as bad as the disease—death of the cell. But it doesn't work that way and Samuel hypothesizes that the double strand on the viral-RNA is what stimulates kinase enzyme production. The kinase blocks production of the initiation complex of chemicals around the double-stranded RNA, but has no effect on the single strand of cellular-RNA. The cellular-RNA creates an initiation complex of tightly formed genetic strands; the viral-RNA can't. So, when the second enzyme floods the area, the cellular-RNA is protected by its circle of strands, like a pioneer inside a circle of conestoga wagons. The viral-RNA, though, remains naked, and an easy target.

A different picture of interferon's abilities comes from Dr. Robert Friedman of the National Institute of Arthritis, Metabolism, and Digestive Diseases. In studies with a virus that induces animal tumors he found that interferon didn't stop creation of viral proteins, but did rob them of their effectiveness. "We can show," Friedman says, "that the virus is being made, but it is not released from the cell surface." Even when the virus was released from an infected cell, it seemed incapable of infecting new victims; the interferon had rendered it useless. Friedman believes interferon-induced changes in the cell surface are what make the viruses impotent.

Ion Gresser, an American working at the Institut de Recherches Scientifiques sur le Cancer in France, found that some interferon effects may be modulated by specific virus-fighting genes in the cell. Working in an area pioneered by Jean Lindenmann, he studied the actions of a particular gene in mice, which he called M_x, that greatly influenced interferon behavior. He concluded that: "the resistance gene can be envisaged either as modulating the antiviral state induced by interferon or as coding for an antiviral mechanism activated by interferon . . . it might be speculated that the seemingly nonspecific antiviral state generally observed in interferon-treated cells would be composed of a multitude of specific antiviral mechanisms, each of which might be coded for by a unique resistance gene."

In other words, interferon might unleash a different fighting gene for every different kind of virus, and perhaps in the presence of cancer as well.

The workings of interferon excite scientists because they afford a view of a whole new system of bodily self-control. Never before has anything been found to work this way. But the most intense excitement in the field has focused not so much on how the potent protein works, but where and on what. The most revered speculation and study have centered on the heart-racing possibility that interferon can control—maybe even eliminate—many kinds of cancer.

chapter 2

INTERFERON VS. CANCER

2

Can interferon cure cancer?

The question, surprising as it may seem, is meaningless. Despite the fact that the phrase "cancer cure" has been tossed about in magazine and newspaper articles for years, it doesn't make any genuine, scientific sense.

A popular metaphor for the elusive cure for cancer is "magic bullet." Where is the magic bullet that will zap cancer without harming any normal body cells? It's an evocative image, reminiscent of the Lone Ranger and the kind of medicine practiced on Star Trek. But, like them, it is the stuff of dreams.

What good, after all, is a magic bullet if you don't have a target to aim it at? Can a magic bullet be effective against a swamp? Can it kill a beast with 200 heads and 200 hearts, all different and independently functioning?

There can be no single cure for cancer because there is no single cause for cancer. In fact, strictly speaking, cancer is not a specific disease. It is a sprawling family of altered body states whose members demonstrate so many different traits, backgrounds and behavior patterns they scarcely seem related. The only property they all share is the phenomenon of unchecked cell growth and the loss of cell differentiation.

The hope for a cancer cure has been linked with the famous, successful searches for polio and infectious disease eliminators. It is a false comparison. Polio is a single, definable, recognizable disease with a discoverable cause. The cause is an agent foreign to the body. The body wants to eliminate this invader and the vaccine helps it do that. Cancer, on the other hand, grows from such various and obscure roots that we can barely find them, let alone attack them. And, more importantly, all of these causes lie within the body itself. Our own bodies, and not the direct intervention of foreign agents, create cancers. Cancer is not so much a disease as an altered state of existence. Parts of our body simply adopt different rules for functioning and the rest of our system seems unwilling or unable to do anything about it. Some doctors even feel that in cancer, our cells return to the wild growth state of the fetus. While this is necessary in the womb, it becomes fatal in adulthood.

Cancer doesn't even have a discreet starting point. You can't say that a person didn't have cancer on Monday and did on Tuesday. It develops so slowly and so intricately—it is so intertwined with the normal bodily functions of cell division and growth—that separating the time when a victim becomes "sick" from when he is "well" is virtually impossible. If we can't separate well and ill, we can hardly expect to have a clear line between cured and not-cured.

To talk reasonably about the ability of any medication, including interferon, to combat cancer, we must think in terms of "treatment," rather than cure. The true question for any new cancer drug is not whether it can cure, since this is by definition impossible to determine, but how well it treats the patient and condition.

Now, the word treat has two sides to it. First, how rudely does the drug treat the cancer? Does it make the tumor shrink? Does it reduce the number of cancer cells in the system? Does it check the spread of cancer colonies to other parts of the body, a process called metastasis? Does it slow the tumor's growth rate? Does it maximize the body's ability to fight off the cancer or the side-effects of the cancer?

Secondly, how gently does it treat the patient's body? Does it make the patient suffer vicious side effects, or is one left relatively free of discomfort? Are normal cells attacked along with the cancer or are they allowed to function in peace? Does the treatment permanently weaken the body and cause deterioration that will last forever, even if the cancer is controlled? Does the treatment bring the patient added comfort and ability; does it positively prolong life or does it merely elongate the period in which one must endure indignity, discomfort, pain, and disintegration?

Existing cancer treatments get fair marks on the first question, but utterly fail the second question. Chemotherapy treatments are toxic; they kill normal as well as cancer cells, as does radiation. The side effects are sometimes horrendous, making periods of treatment more troublesome for patients than the effects of the disease itself. Many negative effects are permanent, some are disfiguring. These treatments have become increasingly effective over the last few years at controlling the course of cancers. Most cancer patients live longer today than they did a decade ago. Five-year survival rates, the arbitrary cure level accepted in cancer work, are up across the board. But the treatments have left the public depressed and dissatisfied, because their toll on the patient is so devastating and obvious.

That is why the emergence of interferon was met with such enthusiasm by researchers, funding organizations, the press, and the public. Interferon is not a chemical poison and it isn't radioactive.

"Interferon opens up a new form of cancer treatment which is nontoxic. There is no nausea, no vomiting, no diarrhea, or other side effects of chemotherapy. In addition, this material prevents viral infections in our patients. This is crucial since the majority of cancer patients die of infections, many of which are viral. As an antiviral drug only it would be important to develop for cancer patients. We also need to see if interferon could prevent cancer in people at high risk," according to Dr. Mathilde Krim of New York's Sloan-Kettering.[1]

In tests with animals and humans interferon has shown anti-tumor potency on a par with or superior to existing treatments. And it offers potential benefits today's treatments don't have.

Interferon is a natural product produced by our own bodies. In cases of virus attack, it differentiates precisely between infected cells and normal ones. Since it works on systems, not specific causes, it fights well against all viruses. Could it also differentiate between normal cells and cancerous ones? Could it attack the basic systems of cancer instead of the divergent causes of specific malignancies? Is it possible that our own bodies make a substance that fights off all cancers and doesn't ruin our systems?

WHAT WE KNOW ABOUT INTERFERON'S ANTI-CANCER ABILITIES

To best understand the answers to questions of interferon's potential, you first have to see how the notion of interferon as a cancer fighter developed and how the drug is being used today.

The path stretches back to the mid-1960s, when Ion Gresser, a Harvard-trained researcher working at an institute outside of Paris, had a clever idea. Gresser had read about interferon's effectiveness against all sorts of viruses in animals, and he knew from his own work that several cancerous tumors in mice were definitely caused by viruses. (This is not true in humans; no human cancer has yet to be unquestionably linked to a viral cause, though there are suspicions about a few.) If interferon works against viruses, Gresser wondered, would it work against viral cancers in mice? He tried the experiment. Interferon treatments stopped the tumors' growth.

Intrigued, Gresser decided to go one step further. He grafted new tumors onto the mice. These tumors did not have any known viral causes. Would the interferon have any effect on them? It unquestionably did; they shrank significant amounts. Gresser's experiments indicated that interferon did something to tumors in mice, but the study was inconclusive. First of all, was it really the interferon that had produced the shrinkage or something else in the impure mixture he had been forced to use? More pressingly, what could his work say about interferon as a treatment against human cancers?

When Ion Gresser came to Paris in 1965, he planned to spend only two years there; but Gresser has now worked for sixteen years at the small Institut de Recherches Scientifiques sur le Cancer in Villejuif, a small town near the French capital. And for many of those sixteen years, Gresser has spent his time with mice.

"In the years immediately after I came to France I worked to determine the effects of interferon on a virus-induced leukemia in mice. It seemed a natural outgrowth of the work on interferon's anti-viral properties. In 1968, I showed that when you treat mice with interferon you slow down the evolution, the development of the virus-caused leukemia.

"Then, I began asking myself, why does interferon slow down a leukemia? And I thought that maybe it's possible that interferon would also slow down the growth of a tumor if I injected it into mice. So I injected tumor cells into mice, then treated them with interferon and found that even though interferon was only supposed to be an anti-viral substance, it seemed to slow down the growth of the tumor, even when a virus wasn't involved.

"We were the first to show this. It opened up the field of interferon as an anti-tumor treatment. We found with a variety of mouse tumors that if you treated them with interferon daily as if it were an antibiotic, it would slow the growth.

"Now, for the last twelve years, we've been studying just how interferon exerts its anti-tumor effect. We've gone around saying it was a very potent anti-tumor effect and a new way of affecting tumor growth, which should be tried in patients with tumors.

"That, I think, is our primary contribution here. For many

people in the field and outside of it felt that interferon was only an anti-viral substance. That it had no other effect on cells. But we went on and showed over the years that this is not so. We showed that interferon can affect cells in many different ways. Not only can it affect the way they grow, it affects changes in the surface of cells. In fact, it changes the behavior of cells.

"I think the nature of the changes interferon creates in cells varies with the tumor and with the patients. Trying to determine which effects are predominant is a sterile discussion; it's like asking where do you want to live, Paris or London? They're both fine places for different reasons.

"What I mean is, let's say you have two women with breast cancer. It is known that without any treatment at all, their tumors will progress at different rates. The way the tumors will evolve will be different. In the same way, it's turning out, treatment is variable, too. Some patients respond well, others don't respond at all. Nobody can really predict the effects yet. We don't know what the variables are; there are too many unknowns."

The researcher who felt compelled to challenge the questions Gresser had raised despite the woeful lack of knowledge was Dr. Hans Strander of the Karolinska Institute in Stockholm. Strander had received his Ph.D. with Kari Cantell, the Finn who produced virtually all of the world's meager supply of interferon, so he was familiar with the protein's early history. Back home in Sweden, Strander, who is also an M.D., heard about Gresser's experiments and those of Kurt Paucker in 1962 that also demonstrated anti-tumor properties of interferon in animals.

Out of scientific curiosity and compassion, Strander got some interferon from Cantell and gave it to a patient with a cancer called osteogenic sarcoma whose tumor was huge and beyond the help of any other treatment. The patient had already suffered amputation because of this virulent bone cancer. The next stage would have been a rapid spread of the condition to his lungs and eventually death.

Working with the extremely impure biological "soup" Cantell produced, with no idea of what a proper dosage should be, Strander figured that at least interferon wouldn't hurt the patient. To his surprise, after several weeks of interferon treatment, the patient's tumor had not come back; it hadn't spread to the lungs.

When word of the startling development seeped into the Swedish medical system, other doctors began referring their osteogenic sarcoma patients to Strander. He began treating them with interferon, at first without any overall plan, then as part of an informal study of the drug's effects. Eventually Strander treated twenty-eight sarcoma victims in this first series of human interferon treatments. Two-and-a-half years after the interferon therapy, 64 percent of the patients were alive and free of metastases, compared with an overall rate for Sweden at the same time of about 30 percent.

The most modern and massive forms of chemotherapy had managed to achieve similar survival levels, but Strander felt that his patients overall seemed healthier and stronger and happier than chemotherapy recipients. Still, his study was so small, so informal, and so uncertain in its results that it proved little. It did, however, deepen and broaden the scientific speculation Gresser had begun.

The strength and weakness in the work of Hans Strander was his high regard for individuals. Strander took the leap forward into use of interferon in humans because the plight of sarcoma victims in his hospital touched him so deeply. This cancer didn't strike the elderly; it struck teenagers, apparently triggered by the sudden spurt of bone growth that accompanies puberty. Because of the cancer, strapping young men were disfigured by amputation. Quite often it led to a swift, painful death.

Rather than give up on these youngsters, Strander felt compelled to try anything—even untested interferon. His positive results created the first flurry of serious interest in the protein as a cancer fighter. But his regard for the individuals he treated made it impossible for him to refuse to give interferon to anyone. His studies had no control patients who received placebos. And both he and his subjects knew full well that they were working with something new and potentially earthshaking. Their psychological lift may have affected their response.

The upshot was that scientific purists riddled his study as being basically worthless. Strander himself, however, remains firmly convinced that interferon works and admits that his informal study has shortcomings other scientists must make up for in their own work.

"In our first thirty-four cases treated with interferon, only half as many patients developed metastases as might have been expected, and they survived longer. Some scientists, understandably, objected that we had used historical controls—that is, case histories of past patients. Now we have added some contemporary controls and I think the results are turning out to be more acceptable."

Strander has also made small tests with Hodgkin's disease and myeloma, in addition to his startling findings about the cancer-like papilloma wart. How this came about was fortuitous:

"There was some trepidation at the beginning, of course. And some surprises. One of the first persons I injected with interferon was a young woman with plantar warts on her feet, which she had had all her life. They completely disappeared. But when we stopped giving her interferon, they came back. Now, one cannot go around giving constant doses of interferon to keep away common warts.

"But there is one type of wart—a non-malignant virus-caused papilloma—that afflicts children in a most distressing way. These growths are not cancer but they could easily kill. They fill up the whole larynx so that the child can barely speak or breathe. And the only treatment is surgery. The papillomas have to be cut out again and again. One of the children I saw had already undergone more than one hundred operations. I know of some seven cases where the use of interferon has cleared up these growths. They do come back again, but repeated courses of interferon are infinitely easier on a child than repeated surgery."

"To summarize," Strander says, "one could say that there is an effect of interferon on many tumors, but we don't know how strong the effect is compared to treatments available already and also how that effect is generated within the body. We are hampered by having very little interferon so that we cannot test as we might otherwise. If our supply were greater we could produce results of greater solidity."[2]

Strander announced his results, tenuous as they were, at an International Conference on interferon in 1975. In the audience at Rockefeller Institute was Dr. Jordan Gutterman of the M.D. Anderson cancer center in Houston, Texas. "That is where I first heard the results, and I was very intrigued not only by the results Dr. Strander was achieving but about the whole possibility of using the various interferons in cancer patients. Here was a nontoxic substance, a natural substance, that not only stopped the growth of viruses but stopped the growth of cancer cells, and it seemed that his material was worthy of further work. The problem was simply one of money."[3]

Money. If interferon had been more widely available and less expensive to produce, it would have followed the traditional path of scientific discovery. Once initial indications of potency had been uncovered, massive studies would have been undertaken. Thousands of patients would have been given the drug at all sorts of dosages, and under all kinds of conditions to see what worked best. Pilot projects with virtually every form of cancer would have been undertaken. Out of this flood of information, a full picture of interferon's abilities would have emerged in just a few years. But this was not the way it would work.

Treating a single patient with interferon costs thousands of dollars. Creating a large study would require incredible amounts of money. Gutterman, despite his keen interest and important position, couldn't garner enough money for a big study. But he did convince medical philanthropist Mary Lasker to provide enough backing for initial tests.

These tests, in which five of nine women with advanced breast cancer showed improvement, were the precursors of the major studies that would bring interferon into the limelight. As one of the earliest testers of the drug, Gutterman has a deeper perspective on its performance and possibilities than most others.

He works in a small lab in the oldest section of the rambling M.D. Anderson Hospital and Tumor Institute. His office is jammed with glasses in bewildering array. Beakers, jars, retorts, flasks, dishes, pipes and bubbles vie for space on his tall, narrow shelves with a spooky phalanx of electronic gadgetry and intricate tangle of rubber hose. Yet, in the midst of this impending chaos, Gutterman—with his staff of three assistants, six nurses and two secretaries—calmly manages to carry on some of the most important research in clinical biology today. His hometown magazine describes him as being like "a juggler in the middle of his act, with hoops all hovering in the air, he pays attention to each detail only as long as he has to and then shifts his attention elsewhere."[4]

Like a wound spring, Gutterman bounces around, speaking quickly, shifting topic suddenly. Only when he talks about interferon does he slow down. Here he can focus his attention for hours and talk with genuine, if cautious, enthusiasm:

"It looks like interferon does have the capacity to induce the regression of tumors, and it probably has at least three mechanisms of action. First, it has a direct effect in terms of stopping or slowing down tumor growth by a variety of different biochemical actions.

Second, it has this very interesting property of immunomodulations primarily to stimulate the body's immune response (the body's way of fighting off disease) so it can activate components of the body's own defenses against the cancer. Third, which may not have anything to do with its anti-tumor effect, is its anti-viral effect."

Gutterman reflects on the origins of his study, which created the modern interferon boom: "We got a small amount of interferon from the National Cancer Institute last February. We've tested about twenty-five patients in all. But we saw enough to know that there are indications among those patients that we can induce some degree of regression of tumors suggesting that even in the small doses we used there was enough potential to warrant further investigation. In the next series of experiments we will be using the same type of interferon but in a larger dose and on many different types of tumors to solidify our results.

"Two million dollars is really quite generous as research grants go," Gutterman points out. But he adds that developments soon will, hopefully, make such enormous outlays for interferon unnecessary. "Scientists are coming up with ways to synthesize the drug, and it looks like we're going to have a very pure form of the drug soon. Because the interferon itself is nontoxic, this will allow us to up the dose."

One member of Gutterman's staff has said, "Jordan's definitely got something, but he doesn't have a cancer cure. What interferon may represent is a part of a multi-component cancer drug that's still some years down the line."

Gutterman essentially agrees. "Obviously," he states, "we've been elated at the response in advanced cancers for whom all treatment possibilities had been exhausted, but the hope is to show just how good it (interferon) will be in earlier disease.

"One other fact that is very important to understand is this: no one, I think, right now would imply that interferon *alone* would have a major impact on many of these tumors. But the fact is we've had very interesting effects and very interesting responses—eight partial remissions and complete remissions in patients who are resistant to a whole series of chemotherapeutic compounds. So it is very clear to me at least that adding interferon to conventional chemotherapy, at the minimum, would be something of great excitement for the future.

"In any case," he says, "it definitely is not going to be just one more treatment. Interferon opens a whole new concept in treatment—using the body's natural substance.

"I think in the next year or two as we begin to work with all three of the interferons and come to understand them better and perhaps use them in combination, we're going to see even greater effects. We have a lot of work to do to understand how to use them, and then finally we have to integrate interferons—the whole field—with conventional therapy. Because we are seeing results in patients totally resistant to chemotherapy, I think that at the very least the whole system of interferon will be an important addition to the therapeutic approach in cancer. Of course, being an anti-viral agent, it has the advantage of probably protecting against various types of infections.

"I think the final message must be that we now have biological agents that seem to induce regression of cancer, which I think is a new idea. The biological agents that we've worked with over the years have not been able to do this. I think this will open the door to other possible biological approaches. There are agents, of course, that can affect differentiation. I fully expect over the next ten years that a variety of substances will be coming along that will have very interesting potential, but it's going to take a lot of hard work."

Today Gutterman feels that, "on a scale of one to ten we've only achieved the first step." However, "the explosion of knowledge that's occurring is phenomenal," he says enthusiastically, "and interferon is only one of the many avenues of treatment. It's exciting that there is an anti-viral—maybe an anti-cancer substance—that's made in the body that's now being scaled up and purified in the lab."

More cautiously, Gutterman notes, "It took 194 years to treat scurvy, years and years to treat smallpox, and it's going to take a long time and a lot of money to cure cancer. We'll keep nipping away at it, but cancer is a hundred different diseases, and we can't do it overnight."

As Gutterman was performing his early tests, other researchers were, indeed, nipping away at the enigma of interferon. Dr. Thomas G. Merigan of Stanford found tumor shrinkage in four of seven patients with a particular kind of lymph system cancer. Dr. David V. Habif of Columbia reported significant tumor shrinkage in six women with metastatic breast cancers.

Through the 1970's, pressure for major studies of interferon grew. Small, anecdotal studies were raising ever more interesting possibilities, but they weren't large enough to prove anything. Their implications, however, were striking. Interferon seemed to have some effect against both fast- and slow-growing cancers, which most other treatments don't. It appeared to have few side effects. Some of the trial patients had undergone reversals of their cancers so startling as to be almost unbelievable.

But none of this amounted to very much scientifically. It could all be a fluke. Despite the expense, a major study of interferon would have to be undertaken.

In 1978, Gutterman went to the American Cancer Society with a most audacious request. He proposed that the society buy $2 million worth of interferon for a 100-patient study of just what the drug accomplished. And he wanted an answer fast. Dr. Frank J. Rauscher, the Society's director of research, was of two minds about interferon's worth, but his proposal review committee was heavily in favor of the study and of getting it started as quickly as possible. So, Rauscher dipped into the society's special $5 million fund for best bets that might bring benefits to cancer patients quickly.

The result was the largest grant in Cancer Society history—$2 million—enough money to buy interferon to treat 150 patients at nineteen different institutions. Four types of cancer were chosen that had shown some response to interferon in the past: breast cancer, non-Hodgkin's lymphoma, multiple myeloma, and melanoma.

It was this decision that brought interferon into public awareness. Suddenly the obscure drug was splashed all over front pages and magazine covers. Interferon researchers were buttonholed by reporters, and asked questions they couldn't begin to answer. The ACS decision, a first step in the determination of interferon's effectiveness, was taken as a rock–solid endorsement of the drug's curative powers. But scientists at the time really had no idea what interferon could do. They needed all that money—and some time—to find out.

In addition to experimental time, interferon research required support. Even in 1978, when the ACS weighed in with its checkbook, no one fully understood what interferon did inside the body and precisely what it was made of. Such information was vital for creating effective experiments and for understanding both positive and negative results. Clinically testing interferon without knowing how it worked or what it was made from was like test-flying a jet without understanding what made it fly. If it crashed, you couldn't hope to explain why.

Much of the work at supporting interferon study was shouldered by Dr. Mathilde Krim. In 1974, by sheer force of will, she talked the prestigious Memorial Sloan-Kettering Institute in New York into holding a seminar on interferon's possibilities. She, personally, was convinced that something was going on in interferon experiments that held great promise for cancer treatment, but the leaders at Sloan weren't so sure. In order to sway them, Krim set up her seminar.

The ploy worked. After hearing what was said at the symposium, the Sloan allowed Krim to set up a small Interferon Evaluation Program and lab. Rather than working with patients, Krim's outfit would study the interferons themselves.

What did they do to cells? How were they built? What activated and deactivated them? Much of our basic knowledge of interferon today comes from the studies done in Krim's labs. While clinicians were getting ready to test people, Krim was making it possible to interpret their results with some clarity, so that whatever powers interferon demonstrated could be put to practical use quickly.

In mid-1979, just as the interferon bandwagon was beginning its roll forward, U.S. Representative Claude Pepper held a meeting of his House Committee on Aging to discuss new treatments for cancer. This stuffy House meeting room offers as good a place as any to hear what the leaders in the field had to say about where interferon was and where it was headed in the immediate future.

There, Mathilde Krim noted that we must know in full detail what interferon is before we can use it most wisely: "When at hand, such knowledge will make it possible either chemically to synthesize human interferons, which could then be made in unlimited amounts, or to use recombinant DNA technology to insert a gene coding for human interferon in a bacterium or another simple cell, such as can be grown rapidly and inexpensively on a truly industrial scale. Interferon could then be produced very much as penicillin is today, also in virtually unlimited amounts."[5]

And Hans Strander emphasized interferon's special natural potential:

> *Interferon is part of our natural defense system. It can be obtained in mass quantities, concentrated and purified. It can be given to patients without causing serious side effects. It has been shown that interferon therapy can cause regression of human tumors, both malignant and benign.*
>
> *It is my strong feeling that this field should be given financial support for escalation. Much work has to be done on the production of interferon, on its purification, and on the elucidation of its structure, on laboratory effects and effects on animal disease. Extended clinical trials have to be done in order to expand a field which shows great promise for the therapy of malignant disease in man.*[6]

In other words, interferon stands on the brink. A little more supply, a little more knowledge, and a little more testing could bring the breakthrough that is so desperately desired. It won't be the breakthrough of a cure-all, or a magic bullet; it will be the more realistic breakthrough of an effective, wide-ranging, benevolent treatment that could help the lives of thousands.

Interferon has shown clear, convincing evidence of a broad antitumor capability. This power isn't universal. For reasons not yet fully understood, it varies from cancer to cancer and person to person. But, in the words of Dr. Frank Rauscher of the American Cancer Society: "We have never seen a drug that showed so wide ranging a set of effects at so early a stage of development."

"It will slow up the growth of tumor cells and, given enough interferon, it will actually destroy some of the tumor cells, shrinking the tumor, mainly in animal systems, but now confirmed in human systems," states Dr. Samuel Baron, one of the earliest interferon researchers.

In animals, primarly mice, interferon has been shown to be effective at reducing many kinds of tumors. Animal studies are considered, among scientists, the closest we can come to human testing in research. Since animal diseases and responses are analogous to human ones, they give researchers a strong notion of what human potential should be and how it can be tested.

Animals are tested before people because of the obvious safety and cost factors along with time considerations. What's more, animals with shorter lifespans than humans develop many diseases faster than we do: The lifetime course of a cancer can be studied in a mouse during a year, where in a human it would take decades.

Tumors studied in animals include:

- *Experimental and virus-induced tumors.* A host of cancers that rise from viruses have been reduced by interferon treatment in several kinds of animals.
- *Spontaneous tumors.* Mice suffering from naturally caused leukemia and mammary cancers were treated with interferon. In the case of leukemia, interferon therapy resulted in a doubling of life span even if treatment began after clinical diagnosis. Chemotherapy agents don't perform as well when begun this late. At present, Mathilde Krim believes interferon appears to be the most active anti-tumor agent against certain types of mouse leukemia. Mammary cancer treatment brought some increase in lifespan and suppressed side diseases that often complicate the situation.
- *Transplantable tumors.* These are clearly non-virus malignancies, but interferon still had a strong impact on them. After several weeks of interferon treatment in one study, 90 percent of treated mice survived more than six months, while no untreated mice lasted past day twenty-two. In the case of one transplantable lung tumor in mice, interferon slowed the growth of both the initial tumor and metastases. When human cancer cells have been transplanted into experimental mice, they have demonstrated susceptibility to human, not mouse interferon.
- *Chemically-induced tumors.* Interferon stopped tumors resulting from certain carcinogenic chemicals in some mouse experiments.
- *Radiation tumors.* When mice, being treated by radiation were given low doses of interferon, incidences of resulting radiogenic lymphoma went down.

In addition, animal studies have shown that interferon treatment, when blended with chemotherapy or radiation, often produces better results than either therapy by itself. When mice afflicted by a particular leukemia strain were given interferon, no improvement resulted. A chemotherapeutic chemical alone produced 25 percent long-term survival. But the chemical followed by interferon resulted in 70 percent long-term survival rates. And, among survivors, only the animals that had both therapies proved to be totally free of lingering cancer cells.

It worked with surgery, too. Surgical resection of a mouse mammary tumor increased lifespan by 79 percent over untreated mice. Surgery followed by interferon increased lifespan by 215 percent.

INTERFERON'S ACHIEVEMENTS: A CHECKLIST

We have talked some about human interferon studies, but here is a formal listing of the cancers studied so far about which doctors have developed a reasonable amount of information:

- *Osteogenic sarcoma*. An update of Strander's precedent-setting study found that five of ten interferon recipients were still alive and disease-free after five years, compared with five out of twenty-one who didn't receive interferon.
- *Papilloma of the larynx*. These are benign, but cancer-like tumors of the throat. While they aren't cancerous, they can be fatal because they close off the windpipe, choking victims. Traditionally, the only treatment has been messy surgery, and even then the tumors inevitably returned. Strander found that interferon treatments gradually reduced the tumor over several months until it entirely disappeared. When interferon was stopped the tumors returned and when it was started again, they vanished. Patients on a biweekly interferon schedule have had no recurrence.
- *Papilloma of the bladder*. A Danish study treated a small group who suffered these recurring bladder tumors. Under interferon treatment, the growths completely vanished in from two to seventeen months.
- *Multiple myeloma*. A painful bone marrow cancer which stymies the system that manufactures our red blood cells. In a study of twelve patients at Karolinska Hospital in Sweden, the four with extremely advanced disease responded to neither interferon nor to any other treatment. Of eight patients with less critical conditions, one stayed in place, four showed partial remissions, and

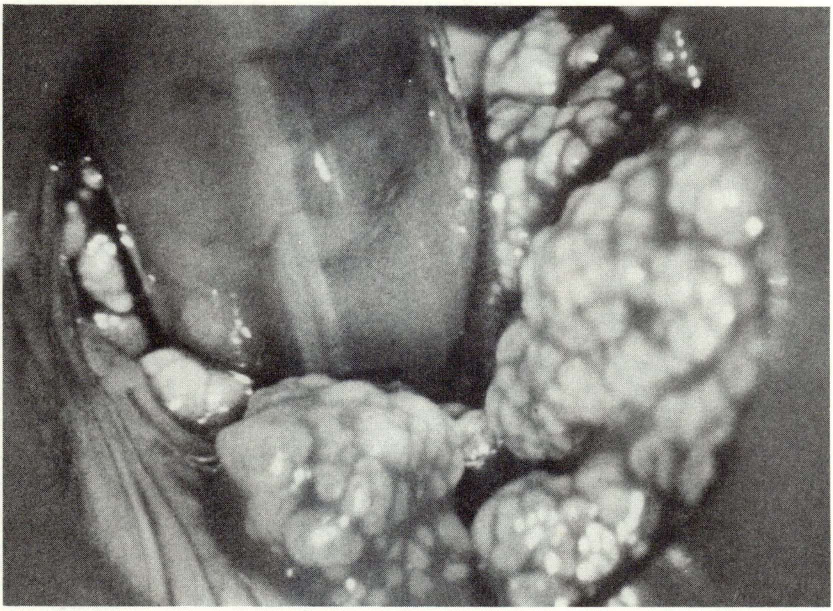

The beneficial effects of interferon can be seen in these photographs of human vocal cords. Above, cancer-like growths before treatment; below, vocal cords after treatment with interferon.

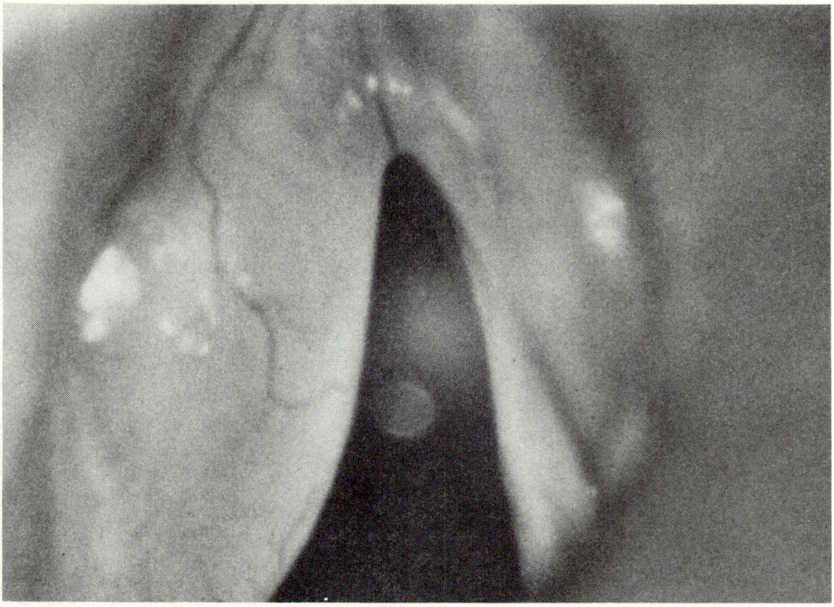

Radiumhemmet/TIME Magazine

three showed complete remissions. Four other patients who had previously had chemotherapy with no effect, included one who achieved partial remission through interferon. Gutterman treated ten cases in Houston and achieved positive responses in six, some of whom had gotten no help from chemotherapy.

- *Breast Cancer.* A Houston study looked at seventeen women whose breast cancer was rather advanced and had withstood all previous treatment. Two doses were used. Five of twelve women receiving a lower dose, and two of six getting the higher amount responded. Regressions occurred in breast tissue, bone metastases, and marrow complications. A few cancerous lesions disappeared. Other studies have achieved similar results.

Studies so far haven't determined just how effective interferon might eventually prove to be against breast cancer. "But that's not the important thing right now," states Dr. Ernest Borden of the University of Wisconsin, who is in charge of part of the testing. "What's important is that we have seen anti-tumor effects with interferon in breast cancer. Interferon is an immunomodulator and so it means that interferon represents another way of attacking tumor cells."

- *Lymphoma.* Dr. Merigan at Stanford has found that interferon generates responses in lymphoma patients. He has gotten positive results with Hodgkin's disease victims, but a known, effective treatment for this disease already exists. The less treatable non-Hodgkin's lymphoma patients responded in four of seven cases. Gutterman tested six lymphoma patients; two achieved more than 50 percent regression, two had lesser remissions, one remained stable and one got worse.
- *Cervical Cancer.* In a Yugoslavian trial, powdered fibroblast interferon was applied through the vagina to thirty-nine women suffering from cervical cancer. All reportedly showed beneficial responses which lasted more than 1.5 years.

Most of the above work was done with human leukocyte interferon, the common form produced by Kari Cantell. At Roswell Park Hospital in Buffalo, New York, studies have been undertaken with fibroblast interferon, the version that comes from connective tissue. Daily injection of the interferon into melanoma, breast, and prostate cancer tumors brought major growth inhibition in about half the cases. Some tumors shrank to one-quarter of their original size within two weeks of treatment.

Lastly, there has been some speculative, but highly interesting results showing that interferon cleans leukemia cells from the system. Although the number of studies is fairly large, the number of people involved is extremely small. In 1980, Dr. Rauscher of the American Cancer Society (ACS) began a worldwide search for interferon recipients. He found 242 people had received the drug, a disappointing number which is the direct result of interferon's incredible rarity. On the plus side, however, 170 of these recipients had shown positive responses to treatment.

INTERFERON'S PRESENT . . . AND FUTURE

In May, 1980, the first preliminary results of the American Cancer Society's interferon tests were announced at a meeting in San Diego, California. A selection from headlines and stories of the event tell the unsettling tale:

> *Experts Downplay Interferon As Cancer Drug*
> *Reports Question 'Effectiveness' of Cancer Treatment*
> *Studies Put Cancer Use In Doubt*
> *Interferon Studies Disappointing*
> . . . *Bewildered* . . . *Discouraged* . . . *Perplexed* . . .

Despite all the exciting work that had come before, the ACS' first studies achieved remarkably mediocre results. "Some significant response" in just four of fourteen patients with multiple myeloma, and partial responses in only five of sixteen breast cancer victims. What happened?

One theory is that a freeze-drying process used to preserve some of the interferon for transport sucked much of the potency from the drug. Swedish researchers recently found that freeze-dried interferon lost 20 to 60 percent of its punch. Much of the ACS supply had been freeze-dried.

Another thought was that, in trying to stretch out the small amount of interferon to the maximum number of patients, researchers had made their dosages far too low. From this point of view, the mere fact that these low doses generated any response was a positive sign.

Whatever the cause, the effect of the announcement was like a bracing shot of cold water in the flushed face of the interferon movement. As sharply as they had trumpeted interferon for months previously, the press blasted the drug's potential. Scientists grumbled about being chastised for failing to live up to expectations they had not done much to raise.

From the pedestal of "cancer cure," interferon plummeted onto the heap of bogus cancer treatments. But, just as the first view was exaggerated, so is the second.

In response to the negative onslaught in the press, Dr. Krim and her staff wrote to the *New York Times* that, however laudable their intent, the articles had "implied fresh doubts about interferon's potential efficacy in human cancer. We attempt here to put this potential in proper perspective because it is the public's will and support that will make further progress possible."[7]

The letter went on to note that interferon used today is less than one percent pure and that supplies are so strapped that experiments cannot be set up as neatly as researchers would like. Given the drawbacks, "the remarkable thing was that under these circumstances interferon should be able to do anything at all."

The core argument in the letter was that interferon hasn't been tested enough yet to be labelled either better or worse than existing treatments. It is more promising because it has shown basic response and remains largely unexplored, but not necessarily better or worse. Only time with increased production and purity will determine that.

The flurry of negative comment in the early summer, however, didn't stop interferon research, and, truly, wasn't justified by events. As the summer progressed, interferon moved back over to the positive side of the ledger of public opinion, though not so hysterically far over as it had once been.

During the summer:

- Shell Oil Company donated $2 million for more interferon purchases, half to the American Cancer Society and half to the Interferon Foundation in Houston. The donation raised the ACS stake in interferon to $6.8 million and was a major step in the Foundation's goal of gathering $20 million for interferon research by the end of 1981.

- The National Cancer Institute committed $9 million for interferon work, signed four interferon production contracts, and began sifting through sixty-three proposals for clinical trials.
- The National Institute for Allergic and Infectious Diseases provided $3.59 million for research into interferon's role versus infections as well as its structure and mode of operation.
- Sloan-Kettering's researchers managed to produce 100 percent pure leukocyte interferon for the first time. It won't be used for treatment, yet, but for study into interferon's structure and operation.
- Production expanded enormously, with ten United States companies jumping into the fray, along with a number of new foreign operations. All of this, of course, is a prelude to the genetic engineering boom that is fast approaching.

Interferon is unquestionably on an upward path toward widespread medical use and acceptance. The disappointment of early 1980 was merely one of the inevitable troughs in any long course. It was as much the outgrowth of problems in cancer testing as in interferon itself.

Despite any temporary setbacks, the quintessential fact that enflames the expanding excitement of interferon researchers and promises a remarkable future for the drug is this: In 220 of the most incorrigible cancer cases on Earth, a messy biological soup that was just one-tenth of one percent interferon was so potent that it shrank or held in check tumors in 172 people.

What on earth could a wallop of 100 percent pure interferon do to an early cancer or the cancerous flotsam left after tumor surgery?

That question won't be answered until late 1981 at the very earliest, and probably not for some time after. But right now researchers have a fairly clear picture of what interferon will be capable of and where it will fit in the scheme of cancer treatments. Keeping in mind that new developments could always alter the situation unexpectedly, the preponderance of feeling in the field today is that:

- Interferon is not the cure-all for cancer, because there is probably no such thing. It will not eliminate all forms of cancer on contact. It will not make every other form of cancer therapy obsolete.
- Interferon is a cancer treatment of enormous potential, having demonstrated more anti-tumor strength at this stage of its development than previous drugs.

- Different types of cancer show different responses to interferon. One view holds that the more environmentally induced cancers show the least response while those that act most like viral infections show the most response, but this hasn't been systematically demonstrated. Some cancers seem fairly resistant to interferon.
- Interferon does, without question, show anti-tumor capabilities, but the precise mechanism by which it works is unclear. Many experts feel that the natural killer (NK) cells do the actual tumor eradication, called into action by the interferon's presence.
- Whatever mechanism is at work, the interferon itself almost certainly doesn't act directly upon the cancer cells. When interferon and cancer cells confront each other in petri dishes, not much happens. The conclusion then is that interferon must stimulate the body to work on the tumor, rather than doing the job itself.
- Interferon has an exciting tendency to work best against tumors when they are in their resting phase. This is in contrast to most anti-cancer treatments, which work best during the tumor's infrequent active phases. Interferon treatments, then, fill a gap left by other cancer treatments.
- Team-ups of interferon and existing cancer therapies seem to work exceptionally well, at least in the laboratory.
- Interferon attacks both primary tumors and metastases.
- Side-effects of interferon treatment do exist, and doctors aren't entirely without concern (see Chapter 6, "The Two-Edged Sword"). However, to date interferon treatment side effects don't seem as painful or as hazardous as those of other cancer treatments.
- Interferon is the first of what will probably be a long line of biological agents—chemicals produced by our own bodies—that will become medically significant over the next few years.
- Patients under interferon therapy are not only aided in their cancer fight, but are protected from viral infections. Often, viral infections brought on by a cancer patient's weakened condition do the actual killing in cancer deaths. Eliminating them, by itself, will increase life expectancy.
- The different types of interferon show different cancer-fighting properties. To some extent they seem to work best against the cells most similar to those they came from. In an extreme example, patients with papilloma were treated with fibroblast in-

terferon; nothing happened. Later leukocyte interferon completely eliminated the tumors.

- There is some indication that the cell surface protective properties of interferon make the spread of cancer through the body harder. Metastases may be a cell surface phenomenon with cancer cells latching onto normal cells and converting them into rogues. The presence of interferon makes this surface binding harder by slowing, possibly even eliminating, metastatic spread.
- No one has any idea why interferon has greater effects in some people than others, just as there is little idea why some people get cancer and others don't. The complexities of personal biochemistry are surely involved but no one knows just how.
- Dr. Lois Epstein of the University of California, San Francisco, has developed a method that potentially could separate out those people whose cancers have the best chance of responding to interferon. She found a way to grow an ovarian cancer in the laboratory, where she could expose samples to interferon. In more than 70 percent of the samples she tried, the interferon shrank the size of the tumor colony.

  "This is of particular importance," she says, "because present supplies are so severely limited. If it would be possible to sort out those patients who would most benefit from those who would not greatly benefit, it would help not only the patients, but would expand the supply of interferon for the entire world."

  She envisions samples of cancers submitted by doctors for testing. If the lab test reveals a high susceptibility to interferon the patient will receive the drug. If the cancer doesn't respond well in the lab, the doctor can try other methods of treatment. In addition, by studying which cancers respond and which don't, researchers may glean a better understanding of just how interferon and cancer interact.
- The most potent anti-cancer interferon is probably the recently discovered Type II immune interferon. Although researchers such as Dr. Samuel Baron of the University of Texas in Galveston have been making immune interferon for testing, there still isn't enough of it available for human testing. If, however, interferon's anti-tumor action derives from the natural killer cells of the immune system, then immune interferon—acting in the system it is most familiar with—could easily outstrip the other forms.

In one early test, small amounts of immune interferon added to leukocyte interferon increased its performance by at least 50 percent.

What, in the end, will interferon's anti-cancer role be? For the next year or two, interferon will remain almost entirely experimental. Genetically engineered interferon is due within the year, as is synthetic interferon made by a complicated process called sequencing. Together, these products will allow for far greater testing. Expanded testing will tell us where interferon is most effective and provide the details about dosage, manner of administration, length of treatment, and so on.

Once this process is complete, interferon can and will be used readily by doctors in their mix of treatments against cancer.

A few cancers—those with viral origins or a particular susceptibility to the drug—will be treated with interferon from the first diagnosis. It will shrink the tumors on its own.

More often, a diagnosis of cancer will be followed by an initial treatment more radical than interferon therapy. Interferon has proven most effective against small tumor burdens; large, well-developed tumors haven't responded very well. As a result, removal of the original tumor through surgery will probably still be the first response to cancer.

In many cases, interferon therapy will begin before surgery and continue afterward, building up the body's defenses against the cancer to a high point just after the offending cell mass is removed. Together, they will serve as a "one-two punch" against the tumor and any residual cells.

Once the tumor is removed, interferon will either supercede or co-exist with chemotherapy and radiation in keeping the cancer away. Since interferon seems to prevent metastases quite well, it should hold a preeminent position in this kind of treatment.

Most likely, when the cancer is diagnosed early and the form of cancer is not particularly virulent, interferon alone will handle the cleaning-up operation. In cases where the tumor is messier, the cancer more advanced, or the chances of spread more ominous, interferon will be used with another method for maximum clout against remaining cancer cells.

Patients who survive a first cancer have a high risk of getting a second cancer; they may receive regular interferon treatments to stop any potential cancer.

Even in cases where no treatment can save a patient's life, interferon will find its uses. It might protect from virus infection and help keep one more healthy and strong so that chemotherapy and radiation can be offered at top levels, allowing the patient to outpace the disease. It will also slow the rate at which an inoperable tumor grows, stretching life expectancy and pushing back the onset of the cancer's worst indignities.

In sum, interferon will certainly become a paramount treatment of cancer. It holds an excellent chance of becoming the principal therapy for keeping cancer patients disease-free once the initial attack has been turned back. For many a cancer sufferer in the years ahead, interferon may represent, literally, an agent that keeps the ravaging condition subdued and allows the recipient to go about life in as normal a fashion as possible. Just as the diabetes sufferer receives daily insulin shots, the cancer-prone victim will get regular interferon treatments.

INTERFERON'S POTENTIAL AS A CANCER PREVENTATIVE

Some interferon researchers hold out hope that the protein may not only work well as a cancer treatment, but as a preventative as well. "Oh, yes," says Dr. Rauscher of the ACS. "There is every reason to hope that if interferon turns out to be an effective therapy for cancer, it should also be an effective cancer preventative. If we had plenty of it—and if it were found safe to take—I can imagine that people with a genetic or familial predisposition to some form of cancer might want to take it as a possible preventative. The same might be true for people who have worked around or have been exposed to dangerous substances, such as asbestos or radioactive materials."

This could turn out to be true, but it raises a peculiar problem: How do you prove something prevents cancer? The disease takes twenty years or more to develop and its appearance is governed by only the most poorly understood rules. We can't yet fathom why eight of ten asbestos workers might get cancer and two won't. We don't know how the innumerable body and environmental factors build on one another to unlease rampant cells. So how do we tell a preventative has been effective?

Let's take the case of a group of high risk printing plant workers. Cancer rates among them are higher than normal. All are given interferon three times a week. In twenty or more years, the entire group dies of natural causes or any non-cancer related accident or sickness. What have we proven? Nothing. Many of those who would eventually have gotten cancer might have died first of another cause. Our evidence is circumstantial and our conclusions are drawn in sand.

Any study that could show that interferon, or anything else, prevented cancer would have to be gargantuan. Whole towns or entire factories would have to be treated and studied for decades. It's a morass, as so much of dealing with cancer is. Indications that interferon might have preventative properties will come, most likely, from animal studies. Once large amounts of pure interferon are available, researchers will treat cancer-susceptible mice with interferon from birth. Since the lives of mice are so much shorter than our own, and so much more easily controlled, we could learn fairly quickly if the therapy has any significant effect on cancer development in rodents. If there is strong evidence that cancer is prevented, it would be an indication that the same might happen in humans; but this would not be absolute proof. Still, it might result in interferon treatment for the groups Rauscher mentions—as long as interferon doesn't seem to effect recipients adversely.

Testing for an amorphous condition like cancer is extremely difficult. In the case of an infection, testing is easy—if symptoms disappear and the infectious agent vanishes from the body, the treatment works. But with cancer, typically, nothing is so clean cut. Even if the early results of the American Cancer Society study had shown that tumors had disappeared from every patient, it wouldn't have denoted a sure-fire long-term treatment. The only way to discover if a treatment will keep cancer away for years is to watch the tested patients for years. Interferon simply hasn't been around long enough to get any long-term picture.

Conversely, it might require months or years of constant treatment for a drug to overwhelm the defenses that the cancer has taken months or years establishing. Again, interferon tests haven't been around long enough to show this. In addition, the supply nightmare has made it impossible for any studies until now to be more than short-term. After a few weeks or months, the researchers literally run out of interferon.

INTERFERON'S GREATEST LIMITATION IN TREATING CANCER: INADEQUATE SUPPLY

It's amazing that interferon has shown some effectiveness in treating so many kinds of cancer, given the relatively meager amount of the substance that is—and has been—available. As a result, interferon's potential may be enormously underrated.

Consider the problem in determining effective dosages. Typically doctors extrapolate from animal studies what dosages might be fatal and then test a huge variety of treatment levels, right up to the assumed ceiling of tolerance. Unfortunately, a study giving patients genuinely massive doses of interferon could wipe out the entire world supply. This means that studies so far have been limited to relatively small doses. They have shown that interferon has some effectiveness against tumors at low levels, but no one really knows what massive amounts of interferon might accomplish.

In early tests of a new potential cancer drug, there is an additional, quixotic limitation. Because it is unethical for doctors to deny patients the best-known treatment, researchers with a new treatment can experiment only with patients who have already received every acceptible and available treatment. Most often, the testers get those patients whose condition has resisted every previous attempt to control it. If the treatment isn't especially effective against the hardiest cases around, it will never have an opportunity to correct milder ones where it may have a greater chance of success. It's as if baseball rules required that a rookie pitcher strike out the all-star team before pitching to journeymen.

Before enumerating interferon's likely capabilities and locating its niche in the cancer pantheon, we should consider another striking conflict looming on interferon's horizon: the question of *double-blind studies*. Traditionally, a drug's effectiveness is proven through such tests in which neither the scientists nor the patients know who is receiving the drug in question and who is getting a placebo. Psychological and unconscious biases are eliminated, so whatever results occur should derive from the medication.

Recently, however, there have been a few problems with this procedure. Lab testing has gotten better and more ingenious. Engineering of medications has grown more sophisticated and human clinical studies have been enormously enhanced by computer statistical models and other technological aids. Today, researchers often know, without question, that a treatment helps patients long before the double-blind stage is reached. With genetically engineered products—by definition, created and extensively tested to produce specific effects—early certainty of effectiveness will grow even more common.

The researcher faces a dilemma. Can one go through with a double-blind study knowing that half the participants will be denied a treatment the researcher *knows* will help them? More to the point, will the researcher be able to find volunteers, willing to gamble their lives on a fifty-fifty chance of getting the treatment they need? Probably not.

Interferon may turn out to be such a drug. The pressure for information has created an explosion of testing. When supplies expand, this search will become still more feverish and wide-ranging. If unquestionable dramatic effects are shown in these tests, who will accept the challenge and risk of a double-blind study? And, if double-blind studies can't be performed, how will interferon—and many other drugs like it—gain official scientific and government acceptance? Quite possibly, the rules of evidence will have to be changed. Findings may have to be submitted to panels of scientists who will determine if the double-blind information is really required, or may be replaced by stages of use documentation, based on accumulating clinical data.

The double-blind bind raises the chance, though, that interferon could get caught in a border war, like many other substances that haven't received the imprimatur of the FDA in the United States. It may become most widely available first in Europe and Central America where rules for human treatment are more liberal. Researchers in the field hope that the rules will be changed before this occurs, but—as anyone knows—the federal government moves as quickly as it pleases, which is generally as slowly as possible.

All this talk about the effects of interferon avoids one central issue, perhaps the focal issue of the drug's ultimate impact on medicine. The manner in which interferon fights cancer excites scientists as much or more than the extent or details of its action. Even though the range of interferon's power against cancer is not yet defined, the method behind the power has opened exciting vistas for treatment.

While other cancer drugs kill, interferon regulates. It does not annihilate cancer as much as it seems to control it. The body's inability to exert reasonable control over cancer cells is what unleashes the disease; and the revelation, through interferon, that natural agents exist in the body which can assume this regulatory role makes scientific palms sweat.

Through interferon it seems that the body, which created its cancer, becomes able to fight back. Interferon raises the hope in researchers that control of cancers by the body's own defenses is both possible and probable. It is not by any stretch of the imagination a goal that has been reached, nor even the designated result of a planned program. It is merely a hope, but a strong and compelling one that brings a second wind to the long struggle against cancer, and offers a promising new road for exploration.

Other cancer drugs are destructive; interferon, while certainly possessing negative side effects, may be primarily restorative, a quantum leap for the better. As Mathilde Krim explains: "It is possible that one way cancer takes hold in the body is to exhaust the normal defenses of our immune systems. In some people these defenses may tire sooner, so they become more prone to cancer. Ordinarily, our natural killer cells can eliminate aberrant growths that begin, but cancer wears them out and they can't stop it.

"Let's take a random number—fifty. Let's say the normal activity of natural killer cells is fifty. But in cancer patients, observations have shown, the level of natural killing is decreased, sometimes to nearly zero, sometimes down to, say, ten. But if you now give this person interferon, his natural killer cell activity will go back up to fifty. Interferon returns the system to its fighting form."

For years cancer researchers have sought a chemical from within the body that could withstand the subtle defenses of cancer. Interferon is the first they have found. They now know that the body is capable of marshalling its resources against this type of scourge. They don't know exactly how it happens. And they don't know how best to translate this knowledge into effective, practical treatment. But researchers do know it's possible. Interferon has shown that cancer may be treatable without radiation and without chemotherapy—some day.

Our understanding and use of interferon is crude today. Our understanding and use of the bodily systems where interferon practices its influence are even more rudimentary. But it's extremely important—both for short-term improvements in cancer and long-term solutions to the enduring enigma of what allows cancer to rampage—that we continue to test and enhance our knowledge. Only then will we be able to control it.

The situation today is similar to the explorations of Lewis and Clark. As they crossed the continent, they found much that they had not anticipated and suffered many twists, turns, and disappointments. But when they reached America's far shore and waded into the foaming waters of the Pacific, they realized that they had found something of incredible importance to the nation—its definition. For the first time the country would know its true parameters.

Lewis and Clark's trip didn't eliminate the problems of the time. Nor did it represent the full utilization of the land they had crossed. Instead, it set the challenge of the times; it pointed the direction for development; it outlined the scope and potential of what lay ahead.

Interferon findings today have done much the same. They have opened the wide expanse of research into the body's own defenses against cancer through the immune system. They have defined the arena in which the next round of cancer control will be fought. They have created the sense that here, indeed, we have found something of incredible, enduring importance.

Now it must be developed, soberly, carefully, and patiently for the greatest benefit to all.

chapter 3

INTERFERON VS. VIRUSES

3

Helen De Rise, an interferon recipient at Sloan-Kettering, received a powerful chemotherapy agent called methatraxate before beginning treatment with interferon. She had to quit chemotherapy, however, because she got chicken pox. The medication so depressed her immune system that she couldn't fight off the childhood infection. It might have killed her.

Most cancer sufferers don't die as a direct result of their tumors; the complications kill them first. And one of the most feared complications is a virus attack. The patient's defenses are weakened by drugs and radiation. The tumor preoccupies the immune responses that occur. The cancer victim is a sitting duck.

This is why the work of Dr. Thomas Merigan may extend the lives of many cancer victims. He is testing the drug's powers against the viruses that plague those who have cancer.

The results are clear: Even if interferon had never shown the slightest effectiveness against tumors, it would still be important for cancer doctors to have. As an antiviral, interferon holds promise for making the lives of cancer patients far healthier, far more enjoyable, and far lengthier as well.

Merigan, head of the interferon program at Stanford University and one of the architects of the American Cancer Society's interferon testing program, first came in contact with the protein in 1962. He was working at the National Institutes of Health in Bethesda, Maryland, assisting Dr. Christian Anfinsen, a biochemist who later would win the Nobel Prize and who now heads the interferon isolating program at NIH. Merigan recalls that he "had become interested in the chemistry of the substance as an important protein made in the body. But I only spent a few weeks on it before I went to work in human genetics at the Palo Alto Veterans Administration Hospital."

He returned to the field, however, to experiment in 1964 at Oxford. There, he and a colleague found interferon in the blood of children who had been given shots of live measles virus. During the period the interferon was in their systems, Merigan found that smallpox vaccine was ineffective. The interferon blocked the second virus.

A decade later, Merigan took a sabbatical in England and worked on the research team that found the first anti-cold effects of interferon. He brought from those tests a strong sense of interferon's potential as a virus fighter. This led him, by a roundabout route, to his work with cancer. "The patient with a malignancy, is doubly vulnerable," says Merigan. "His immune system is already subnormal. It is further suppressed by chemotherapy and radiation. With resistance so low, infections may appear in their most virulent form. They can cause some patients more misery and anguish than tumors do. Many cancer patients die, not of cancer, but of an accompanying infection. One of the worst of these is herpes zoster—shingles.

"Zoster is not only excruciatingly painful, but can endanger the cancer victim's life as it spreads over the body's skin surface and to the viscera as well," Merigan says. "In a series of three trials involving ninety lymphoma patients, we did observe some interferon side effects—fever, for example, and transient bone marrow suppression at the high dosages necessary. But our trials did demonstrate that interferon can prevent the spread of zoster in cancer patients. We now have every reason to believe that there may be a very useful role for interferon in the treatment of systemic viral infections. The same holds true for transplant recipients. They too have had their immune systems suppressed to prevent rejection—and they are vulnerable to infections which perhaps could be headed off by interferon."

Following his work of tying interferon's virus-fighting potential with cancer and other maladies, Merigan turned to the protein's antitumor effects. His tests of a handful of lymphoma patients were among the first and most influential interferon investigations with humans.

"Interferon is unique," he states, "No other natural substance has such broad activity. Being a natural substance, it may have a greater margin of safety. The jury's still out. But anything with this broad amount of activity will find a unique application in medicine."

Merigan is cautious about the findings of his own early studies. "We found that certain tumors appear to reduce in size under interferon treatment, but we know other agents produce the same results." Still, he wrote in the *New England Journal of Medicine* report on his work, "the positive results achieved in viral infections and tumor experiments in animals and the limited human trials so far completed, suggest that (interferon) could be one of the first natural products for use in human medicine, with an effect potentially as great as that of the corticosteroids (such as the pain killer cortisone)."[1]

The role of cancer patients in Merigan's studies points up the important place interferon's anti-virus abilities have in helping cancer patients. Both a cancer victim's disease and treatment lower resistance to viral infections and ability to fight back against them. As often as not, a terminal cancer victim will die from a viral or other complication before the course of malignancy is run. These viral intrusions greatly increase the discomfort, pain, and depression that a cancer victim is prone to. Interferon's anti-viral abilities significantly reduce these complications.

Examples of the beneficial symbiosis between interferon and traditional cancer treatment first came, typically, from Hans Strander and the Karolinska Hospital. During the treatment of cancer patients with interferon, Strander watched for benefits or drawbacks from interferon's other powers. After years with his patients, he became impressed by their freedom from viral infections. For instance, he found that thirty-three of his fifty patients had suffered no overt viral disease and had generated no new antibodies (a sign of hidden infection) during their course of treatment with interferon.

Another study looked at the differences in viral infection between the group of eight cancer patients who lived at home and the rest of their families. The interferon recipients, again, showed fewer signs of virus infection; considering their conditions, they should have shown far more.

One of the most striking cases of how interferon can improve the lot of a cancer victim, apart from tumor effects, comes from England, where Dr. Phillip Gardiner has been using the protein to stave off measles infections in leukemia patients. When a normal child gets measles, it is a bother for parents and a chance for the youngster to spend a week home from school. But with leukemia victims, measles can be deadly. The drugs required to stimulate and maintain remissions in the disease leave children very exposed.

Furthermore, leukemia also makes measles much harder to detect than in normal children. It's not enough to sit back and wait for spots. Sometimes leukemics get measles without a rash showing. In any case, by the time the disease presents itself, the situation is much too developed and dangerous for real hope. The diagnosis must be accomplished quite early.

Gardiner began testing his leukemia patients for measles at the smallest sign of infection. The simple test could reveal in a matter of hours if incipient infection was underway. When Gardiner received a positive result, he placed the child on either interferon or a placebo. The inclusion of a control made the test's findings highly reliable.

All the children who received interferon remained free of measles. One of them, in fact, had never had a measle vaccine, so his body had no antibodies whatsoever against the infection. Yet, when a family member came down with measles, thus exposing him, he did not contract it. A few pre-illness symptoms appeared, and then went away. Mathilde Krim's report on this study states that: "It may be noted that before receiving interferon these children had been treated with various forms of antileukemic therapy. Interferon could then act (effectively) against viruses despite immunosuppression brought on by treatment. The absence of viral disease in these children is in sharp contrast to the general experience that about half of all leukemic children under therapy contract serious viral or other non-bacterial infections and that about 10 percent of them actually succumb to such infections."

Evidence from various studies has grown so strong that many experts feel interferon can provide excellent protection for cancer victims before the appearance of virus infection. They see the likelihood that many cancer victims will receive interferon as a matter of course during their cancer therapy to hold down viruses, keeping the patient as vigorous as possible during whatever other forms of treatment he must face. The elimination of the viral scourge from the host of things cancer patients and doctors must worry about would be a major medical achievement for interferon, even if it never cures a single cancer by itself.

THE NEW "PENICILLIN"

With all the furor over interferon's potential as a cancer fighter, it is sometimes hard to remember that the drug's original prominence was as a virus fighter. Interferon was going to be the anti-viral penicillin that would free humankind from the scourge of myriad virus infections. This promise has been overtaken and overshadowed by the later-blooming, anti-cancer findings, but power against viruses remains the best documented of interferon's abilities.

During the early years of interferon's existence, it was only the anti-viral possibilities that kept experimentation with the protein going. At the time, few people took its anti-cancer potential seriously. But then virus research levelled off for a number of reasons. First, researchers found that interferon was species specific. Vaccines for individual viruses are not species specific; they will act against a virus in many different kinds of animals. This means that the virus material can be grown in animal cells. Scientists can choose the cells that work best in the lab and use them to incubate huge batches of material that can be fashioned into vaccine that works in humans.

When interferon was first discovered, scientists hoped that it offered a similar option. It was the first agent they'd ever seen that attacked all viral infections at their roots—the cell. They saw it as a vaccine against *all* viruses, not just one. But species specificity made this impossible. Human interferon, it turned out, had to be made from human cells, which were hard to come by and expensive to work with. Many researchers were discouraged enough by this finding to drop interferon from their plans. In any case, the severe supply shortage that persisted for more than a decade drastically limited human experimentation.

Even when the supply situation improved a bit, virus studies suffered. When interferon's anti-cancer potential became a more acceptable concept, new amounts that became available went to the more prestigious cancer work, rather than the virus studies.

More than vanity or politics dictated this allocation of the limited resource. Ethics require scientists to throw most of their effort behind research with the greatest potential benefit. In the case of cancer, the benefits would far outstrip those obtained by limiting viral infection. Viruses tend to be fatal only to the weak, old, or allergic. Most viruses are self-limiting; that is, they peter out on their own after a given length of time in the body. While some viral diseases are fatal, the greater risk lies in cancer, and the weight of research must rest there.

Knowing how desperate researchers have been to get interferon for the paramount cancer tests, you can imagine how sparse the supply has been for virus work. "As long as interferon remains so scarce," states Kari Cantell, "we will have trouble allocating it wisely. For example, we know that interferon is effective against the herpes eye infections, which cause blindness in many of their victims. Suppose there are 100,000 people with such infections and we could treat them all with existing interferon supplies. Is that what we should do with our supplies—or conduct trials on a few hundred cancer patients? This is the kind of ethical dilemma we will continue to face until we get more interferon."

Despite these problems, a small but steady body of evidence on interferon's ability to fight virus has been built up over the years, resulting in a picture of the protein's anti-viral effects that is much clearer than the view of its potency against cancer.

As early in the drug's history as 1960, Britain's Medical Research Council and a trio of English pharmaceutical companies joined forces in an attempt to find out just how good interferon might be as an anti-viral agent in humans. First, they had to overcome the problem of finding or making interferon that worked safely in humans. Burroughs-Wellcome began the search for this, eventually creating a manufacturing process that is utterly distinct from that of Kari Cantell's historic factory in Finland. The researchers' other consideration was how they could set up experiments that would show something useful.

Viruses are a problem to test. Since most of them are self-limiting—they go away in their own time—the mere fact that a virus disappears in an experiment doesn't prove anything. Neither does the absence of infection, since people successfully manage to resist viruses on their own every day.

A lot of thought and planning went into the first anti-viral test. The test had to be fast, decisive, and controlled; it couldn't leave any part of the results to chance. What the testers came up with was a plan to challenge one spot on the body first with interferon, then a virus in quick succession.

This 1961 experiment used monkey interferon, a substance closest in structure to ours and more available for testing. It was injected into the upper arms of volunteers who had never been exposed to or vaccinated against smallpox. For control, a placebo was injected into another spot. The next day, vaccinia virus was placed into both injection locations. If the virus "took" on a site, as a vaccine takes and causes a small reaction in patients, a small lesion would appear. If the interferon blocked the virus's ability to establish itself in the body, nothing would show up on the surface.

The team found that lesions showed up on thirty-seven of thirty-eight control spots and only fourteen of thirty-eight interferon injection sites. The difference was far greater than required to show an interferon effect.

The test was a good one because it gave the experimenters their best chance of getting a positive response. The interferon's effect was locally concentrated and the same cells that had been bombarded with interferon one day got the virus the next. If interferon couldn't protect cells under these coddled conditions it couldn't protect them at all. Once the results were obtained there could be no question that interferon reacted against viruses in people.

But the next step in the process proved much trickier. How well did interferon work in a more normal situation, where all the cards weren't stacked in its favor? Trials in 1965 and 1970 in which interferon was tested against respiratory viruses came out negatively. This was probably because the dose of interferon was just too small to overcome the natural protection of the lung's foreign chemicals. But at the time, the results sent scientists off on a wild goose chase for an alternative way to test interferon.

Since interferon from a source other than the patient didn't appear to have a potency comparable to the patient's own interferon, how could researchers induce the patient to create more of the protecting agent naturally and inside the body? A long series of unfortunate experiments followed. They determined that the part of a virus that goaded interferon production most was the characteristic double-strand viral-RNA. Unfortunately, injections of raw, double-stranded RNA proved to be less effective in animals the more they resembled humans, and the treatments demonstrated disturbing toxic side effects in human volunteers. Frustrated, researchers looked back at applications of foreign interferon as the only alternative they had. In the meantime, Kari Cantell had devised his production method for true human interferon, so experimenters actually had a more pure material with which to work—though not much of it.

The big step forward came in 1972. The Medical Research Council used some of Cantell's interferon for a major, controlled study of interferon against an all-star team of flu and cold viruses. Subjects were given interferon or a placebo and then exposed to the virus under windy, cold conditions that were likely to make them contract an infection.

One virus after another proved itself victorious. Interferon didn't seem to have much effect at all. Then the researchers tried Rhinovirus 4, the instigator of a severe form of head cold. Massive doses of interferon were given as nasal sprays, and the colds disappeared. For the first time, it had been shown that interferon could reduce the impact of a virus cold infection. This achievement was made sweeter because test subjects showed no serious side effects from the treatment.

Joy at the proof was tempered somewhat by the realization that this medicine couldn't be utilized regularly or routinely. There wasn't enough of it to go around the lab, let alone the country. And every squirt of interferon nasal spray cost $1000; even a pasha might balk at paying those prices to dry up a stuffy nose.

Still, the potential for interferon use in virus infections could be seen. And the positive results in England energized a continuing round of studies with many different viral diseases that has yielded a continuing flow of indications that interferon is almost universally effective against them. Not one of these studies pushed interferon ahead to the point where it was unquestionably the best drug to use against a given virus, but they set the stage for later, more specific findings.

Some in the field feel that this steady, clear progress in small viral studies kept interest in interferon alive until the cancer establishment discovered it. These early researchers state that without their interest in holding off infection, interferon might have vanished before its cancer potential was ever realized.

"Interferon is where it is today because of the National Institute for Allergic and Infectious Diseases' belief in it, early on, when the cancer people weren't interested," claims Dr. George Galasso, who championed interferon in the early days. "Since 1969, we put $1 million a year into interferon research. That's not a lot, but it's had to come out of our hide. We've got it up to $3 million this year, but it's a very tough struggle. I'd like to put more into virus studies, but we can't.

"So suddenly there's this big furor over interferon, and I'm pleased with it, because cancer research seems to have more sex appeal for the public and for Congress, which is what counts. But research in infectious disease is getting short shrift, and it doesn't deserve to."[2]

Interferon received early attention as an anti-viral drug because the need for one was so great. Vaccines against specific viruses worked, but with serious limitations. The slightest change in the form of a virus and the vaccine became totally useless. If a flu strain mutated while it was spreading through the population—a common occurrence—all the expensively-produced vaccine could be tossed down the drain; it is only effective against the original form of the infection. Interferon, on the other hand, demonstrated an ability to fight a virus despite any and all transmutations in form. Amazingly, even artificial viruses specifically created to circumvent interferon failed, and were checked by the powerful protein.

In addition, interferon's anti-viral action seemed less fraught with consequences than vaccines. Vaccination involves flirting with an infection in order to hold off a more passionate encounter later on. The vaccine contains dead or dormant strains of the virus. When they are injected into the system, they create antibodies to the virus. Later, when the natural virus shows up, the antibodies will attack it before it can establish itself in the system. But filling a vaccine recipient with viruses obviously carries a risk that a mild attack of the disease will occur. Thus, the reactions to flu and measles shots. In the case of milder viruses, which don't kill most victims, doctors wonder whether giving patients a preventive pre-attack is worth the risk, expense, and bother.

Moreover, some viruses have simply eluded science's ability to create vaccines for them; yet they respond to interferon. These include some of the most dangerous and destructive of the lot: Respiratory viruses kill some 10,000 children a year. Echoviruses lurk behind meningitis outbreaks and childhood paralysis. Coxsackie viruses carry with them complicating, debilitating respiratory epidemics.

There are individuals for whom a vaccine can be deadly and a typically innocuous virus infection even deadlier. They are the immuno-incompetent, people whose bodies can't shake off infection through the ordinary channels. Placing a virus in their system could kill them as could any spontaneous viral infection. Medicine requires something that will protect these most exposed individuals.

Time is also a crucial factor in arguments for interferon. Many virus infections display similar symptoms. In a strong individual with no complications, doctors may have time to sort through lab cultures to find exactly which virus is at work and to formulate a vaccine. But when patients are old, weak, or particularly vulnerable, the doctor may not have time. As a report on anti-viral interferon states:

> *Many viral infections display a similar symptomatology, and the precise identification of the viral etiological agent is often difficult and time-consuming. Therefore, it is important that an antiviral agent with a broad spectrum of antiviral action be available, to allow treatment to be begun before the causative agent can be specifically identified. Thus, any nontoxic agent which could be effective in the prevention or therapy of a broad range of viral infections would contribute substantially to the success of other forms of treatment, as well as to better public health. Should such an agent also be effective against nonviral intracellular parasites, its usefulness would be extended considerably. Interferons may represent the broad-spectrum, nontoxic antivirals still missing from the medical armamentarium.*[3]

Interferon, today, is one of three possible approaches scientists can take toward a virus infection. As noted, the first is vaccination (more accurately, immunization): the injection of an attenuated form of the virus to which the organism will then produce antibodies. They, in turn, can neutralize the virus if it appears again in the body. But this requires prior isolation and characterization of the virus in question, a task which has not yet been completed for many pathogens (the various forms of viral hepatitis, for example). Moreover, viruses are often so many faced and apt to mutate that a vaccine developed against one type will not protect against related varieties (as in the case of the flu).

The second approach involves introducing into the organism novel drugs of limited toxicity whose selective antiviral effects will nonetheless be relatively large. This approach has had some success, and a series of anti-viral drugs based on this concept are currently being tested. An additional strategy in this regard is exploiting the biochemical changes associated with infected cells and the use of general inhibitors of RNA, DNA, or protein synthesis that neither can, nor do, penetrate normal cells. While this can reduce virus multiplication, it cannot prevent the spreading of viruses to healthy, neighboring cells.

And then there is interferon, the method which stimulates the body's own first line of defense. It offers the advantage not just of attack, but of protection. It isolates the virus and renders cells nearby impervious to viral spread. Further, because it is a natural substance,

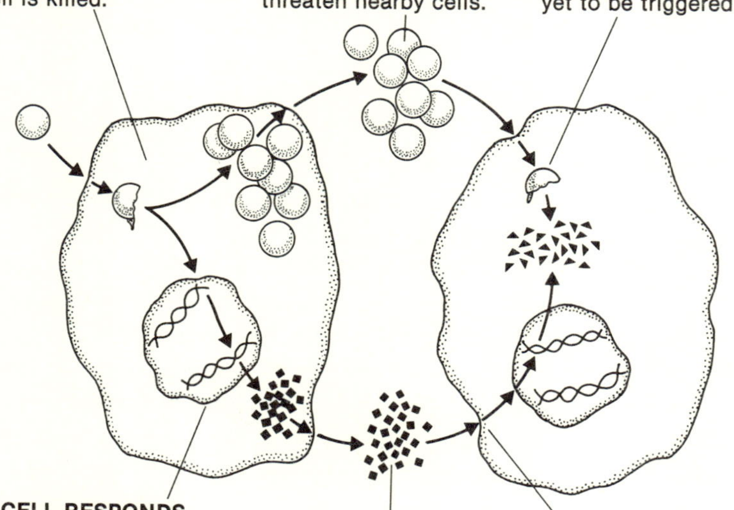

Bob Ritter/The New York Times

it doesn't necessarily carry with it the serious side effects of a foreign chemical drug.

INTERFERON'S VIRUS-FIGHTING ABILITIES

Of the trio of approaches for neutralizing viruses, interferon presents the best theoretical picture for treatment. Researchers have felt a compelling need to find out how well and how many viruses interferon could treat effectively. They focused their work on viral infections for which effective vaccines didn't exist and which created severe problems for the victim. Here is a review of findings on some of those diseases:

Herpes Simplex Keratitis. Herpes is a particularly tenacious virus. It lurks in the nerve centers of victims where it can lie dormant for months. Then, for reasons not yet well understood, herpes will lash out. The attack can hit many different parts of the body. One of the most painful and dangerous forms of outbreak is herpes keratitis, where the virus spurs formation of ulcerated sores of the eyes. These sores aren't deadly, but their repeated appearance and irritation can wear down the area around the eye leading, in some cases, to blindness. Even when their effect isn't cumulatively disastrous, they are exceedingly painful, unsightly, and incapacitating for as long as they last.

Study of herpes keratitis has been responsible for the first indisputable evidence of interferon's anti-viral abilities in both animals and humans. Early tests used rabbits whose tiny eyes had been all but swollen shut by the viral sores. In a startling number of cases, the sores disappeared quickly and totally.

In 1973, at the University Eye Clinic in Freiburg, West Germany, Dr. Rainer Sudmacher set up a full-scale randomized, double-blind study of interferon against keratitis in humans. Forty patients with the ugly sores were split in two groups; half would receive a placebo solution and half a high dosage of leukocyte interferon. The study showed that 96 percent of the interferon-treated patients showed virtually total improvement, compared with 56 percent of the control group.

But this was not the whole story. Other tests using lower dosages given at regular intervals found little effect at all. Eventually, researchers concluded that it took a huge, knockout punch of interferon to overcome the herpes. Steady treatment wouldn't do it. But these studies still left one further question—was interferon merely suppressing the symptoms of the herpes, or would it keep the sporadic reappearances of the problem down? Recurrence has been the Achilles' heel in herpes treatment. No treatment existed that could stop recurrence; it had resisted every chemical and immunological agent doctors had tried.

Studies on this question remain inconclusive. Dr. Mathilde Krim has written: "It took twenty years to achieve these results, and, because the lack of interferon in appropriate amounts makes it impossible to carry out the experiment under optimal conditions, it is still not known whether continuous interferon during the latent period of the infection can prevent its recurrence . . . but it seems quite certain that human leukocyte interferon, given topically at appropriately high concentrations in single daily applications, is effective against active herpes (keratitis)."

Another interesting development in trials of interferon against herpes keratitis is that the protein seems to make another anti-viral agent much more effective against the disease. As Kari Cantell has reported: "Particularly interesting is the combination of interferon and TFT (a chemical treatment) . . . When TFT is supplemented with (interferon treatment), corneal ulcers heal and virus shedding stops significantly faster than when TFT is used alone." Such teamwork could help extend interferon treatments to more patients, and allow far longer treatment periods, helping to clear up the question of interferon effectiveness during latency.

Herpes Zoster. Varicella, the disease most of us call chicken pox, is caused by herpes varicella zoster virus. The same virus also causes the disease zoster—also known as shingles—which strikes adults, opening crops of blisters in patches that follow the courses of the main spinal nerves, sometimes reaching the face and eyes. They are excruciatingly painful and spread as they burst.

Scientists believe that zoster viruses get into the system through the lungs. In children, they initially generate chicken pox. Once that infection has passed, the herpes retreat to nerve ganglia, where they remain until the next eruption, when they slide along nerve fibers to the skin and explode there as ulcers. It can happen at any time after the original infection.

In children, treatment of immune globulin can forestall infection for a brief time, and works well in cases where chicken pox could be fatal to a weakened or sickly child. But in adults, the zoster rampages take place despite the body's existing store of antibodies; and they resist every form of anti-viral treatment. In fact, one treatment that worked in the lab failed to control the outbreaks in people.

Interest in trying interferon against zoster arose because the potent protein was found in cells infected by the virus. Lab studies, moreover, showed that zoster responded to interferon, though not with as much alacrity as other viruses. One of the most important studies revealed that extremely high levels of interferon in the blisters prevented ulceration and the resulting spread of the disease.

These lab indications spurred interest in finding out how well interferon would work against human zosters. Hans Strander discovered in an early study that interferon treatments seemed to help his cancer patients ward off zoster, which often inflicts cancer victims with an additional torment. Building upon this finding, Thomas Merigan at Stanford tried interferon on cancer patients. In a cancer victim whose defenses are already at low ebb, zoster spreads rapidly and can literally make life torturous. Merigan began his treatments within forty-eight hours after the shingles appeared, by which time seven out of nine of his patients had more than 100 open sores spread all over them.

Weakened cancer patients often succumb to the pain and strain of a severe zoster outbreak, but in Merigan's study: "despite their tumors and the fact that they had already undergone extensive cancer therapy and were presumably in a state of immunosuppression, all seven patients survived their disseminated zoster. In none of the patients did it progress to the extent of involving visceral organs, which is otherwise frequent in debilitated individuals." None of the patients showed signs of any toxic side effects or impairment of their body's normal abilities to fight off the disease.

Merigan's study also found that different stages of the disease seemed to respond to different levels of treatment. Visceral spread seemed to respond at relatively low levels of interferon, while spreading under the skin required higher doses for best effect.

A follow-up study by Merigan, using seventeen cancer patients, determined clearly that interferon is effective at preventing the surface and internal spread of zoster. Since most patients die from the subsurface spreading, Merigan's findings indicate that interferon will help weakened patients survive zoster attacks. It also appears to greatly reduce the disease's pain.

Other studies have shown similar results. In Switzerland, for instance, thirty-seven patients, some of whom had cancer, were divided into two groups. One group received interferon, the other a placebo. Researchers concluded that interferon lessened the severity of the disease.

Kari Cantell notes that the positive results against zoster in cancer patients are particularly encouraging because of the depressed immune abilities of people who have gone through chemotherapy and radiation. The interferon effect could be more powerful in otherwise healthy people.

Rabies. When most people think of rabies, the images that come to mind are foaming mouths and the long, painful series of shots that any victim of an animal attack must undergo. The panic following contact with a rabid animal grows from the hideousness of the disease that is caused by the viruses which drive the beast mad. Rabies is a central nervous system breakdown that presently cannot be stopped once it has started. The untreated victim will die invariably, and most unpleasantly.

The only regularly used form of treatment today is the shot series. It is, basically, a massive assault on the body's immune system with a rabies vaccine. Huge and constant amounts of rabies antibodies, hopefully, will prevent any disease from getting started. But the shots are grittingly painful; and they have to be given whenever there is any chance of infection. Of the 30,000 people a year who must undergo this tricky, unpleasant process, many endure it without ever being infected by a rabid animal; their torment is needless.

In animal experiments, interferon and chemicals which induce its production completely protect lab animals challenged with rabies. When given up to three hours after the exposure to the virus, the interferon wiped it out. When administered twenty-four hours after the virus got started, the interferon prolonged the course of the disease, though it couldn't save the animals. Greater amounts of interferon seemed to have greater effects, and interferon administered near the site of the original infection appeared more effective than that remotely administered.

Closer to home, human interferon was given to species of a monkey that had shown sensitivity to it. The animals got interferon injections every other day beginning one day after they were infected with rabies. Some of the animals survived far longer than they should have and others escaped the disease altogether. Testing afterward found that the animals hadn't generated antibody to the infection; it must have been the interferon itself that weakened the infection.

A few experiments have been conducted with rabbits to see if interferon can affect rabies once it has attacked the central nervous system. Three weeks on interferon didn't save any experimental rabbits, but it definitely prolonged the course of the disease. Better understanding of where, how, and how much interferon should be administered could provide more definitive results.

The real teaser in rabies testing with interferon was the case of a Washington D.C. woman who had contracted the disease from a rat bite and already begun to show symptoms. She received interferon therapy, and her symptoms disappeared. While the case of a single individual is not enough with which to draw a conclusion, it is in itself powerful testimony. In the entire history of medical science no other person has ever been reported whose rabies symptoms went away once they appeared. If it was a fluke, it was a monumental one. Dr. Daniel Henley of Memorial Sloan-Kettering Cancer Center is beginning a study of interferon and human rabies in cooperation with the government of Egypt; Egypt is one of the few places on earth where there are enough cases of this rare disease at any one time to field a worthwhile sample.

Respiratory Diseases and Flu. In Russia, comrades with runny noses and itchy throats can buy small spray bottles of a potion the authorities say can help get rid of their symptoms. It's called interferon.

By western standards, this Russian concoction is useless. It is terribly impure, even when compared to the less than one percent purity common today. The amount of interferon is so small that if Cantell spread his supply as thinly, he could treat every Finnish citizen simultaneously. Its effectiveness, if any, is highly doubtful. But it does show that the Soviets have an interest and a certain confidence in the protein's ability to help in cases of respiratory distress.

In reported studies, both Russian and Japanese researchers have found that low-level interferon sprays really do help lessen the severity of flu. Tests elsewhere, however, have had mostly mediocre, inconclusive results.

There are a few shining exceptions, however. One trial used an interferon inducer against the flu-like rhinovirus. Tests showed that virus shedding—a sign of active infection—and other symptoms were blocked, and that interferon seemed to be the cause. Another successful trial used a high-power interferon nasal spray in a controlled situation. Sixteen volunteers received the interferon, and sixteen were given a placebo; the interferon recipients showed less virus shedding and fewer symptoms than the controls. An earlier trial against the same virus at a far lower dosage had proven negative. High-dose interferon treatments may prove far more effective than studies so far have indicated.

In the case of the sixteen volunteers, interferon remained in their systems long enough for researchers to conclude that interferon given as often as time-control remedies would effectively and continuously suppress their infections.

The nose is not the only path interferon can take to the respiratory trouble zones, at least not according to casual information from Hans Strander's cancer patients. He has found that their interferon shots have protected them rather well from respiratory complaints; they have complained much less than their family members. While this doesn't prove that interferon shots are adequate protection from respiratory viruses, it does raise interesting possibilities for future study.

German Measles. This disease, formally known as rubella, puts expectant mothers in fear. The horrendous impact of the virus passes from the mother to the developing child, resulting in birth defects and rubella syndrome fatal in 10 to 20 percent of the cases. Even among babies that survive a rubella-plagued birth, the virus remains. It can be found in the systems of children for years after birth. Many experts feel that this chronic low-level irritation can result in long-term damage in coordination, hearing, and sight.

At first glance, rubella might seem a natural candidate for a vaccine. It is consistent and identifiable. However, there are fears that the virus used in any vaccine might create the same post-birth problems as the live virus. Any fast, potent treatment for rubella in the stricken youngster would be a prize medical discovery.

Interferon's chances of taking the prize remain uncertain. Rubella doesn't stimulate too much interferon production in lab cells taken from fetuses, but it does react strongly against interferon in adult monkey and human cells. As little as four units of interferon have been seen to reduce rubella virus levels by 90 percent. On the other hand, infected baby cells have been found to generate stable knots of impervious, slow-producing virus that low-level interferon treatment can't handle. In the lab, the signals on interferon's worth against rubella have been decidedly mixed.

The first infant treated with interferon, however, showed positive signs. This unfortunate child was born with double cataracts, heart problems, and body malformations. At seven months, his skin erupted in virulent open sores. For seven months he got steadily worse, and his body's signals regarding interferon production were confused. At age fourteen months, though, interferon therapy was started on his skin, and within a week the sores had begun to retreat. By the end of a month, the skin was completely healed. Strangely, the levels of virus found in urine remained unchanged.

Therefore, while interferon might prove an unworkable treatment in infants with rubella troubles, it is by no means certain. At the mother's end of the equation, some researchers have found that certain strains of rubella generate higher interferon production than others, and the strains that generate the most seem to cause the lowest levels of damage to embryos. This raises the possibility that a combination vaccine-interferon therapy could be used in a mother-to-be who has had German measles and doesn't want an abortion. The interferon-producing rubella strains could be used for the vaccine at low risk to the infant. Then, the increased levels of interferon in mother and child might afford a raised level of protection.

Chronic Hepatitis. Interferon's course against this long-term, dangerous liver ailment shows both the potentials and pitfalls in developing interferon as a drug. From the earliest knowledge of the protein, scientists held out hepatitis as a perfect situation for using interferon.

Hepatitis had withstood all attempts to get it out of the systems of sufferers. It was a chronic condition, which offered important research benefits—it wouldn't go away of its own accord before results could be achieved, as many other virus diseases might. Its persistence was well known, so any treatment that broke this established chain could prove itself with few patients, instead of a huge sample. A little interferon given to a small number of victims could, potentially, prove a lot and help a great many people.

All these points were buttressed by the fact that chronic hepatitis is a serious and growing health problem in the world. While most widespread disorders are shrinking, hepatitis is growing stronger. Ten percent of American hospital admissions are for acute hepatitis attacks. Hepatitis virus contaminates one of every 200 blood donors and up to 15 percent of the population of developing countries. Victims are plagued with recurrent attacks for the rest of their lives.

It was natural that hepatitis become the virus of choice of many interferon experiments. Early indications for the protein's effectiveness were not good. Hepatitis patients were found not to have elevated natural interferon levels. In fact, their cells produced less interferon against random viruses in the lab than those of other people. Perhaps the lack of interferon had something to do with hepatitis susceptibility. Or maybe the virus somehow dampened the protein's action—which would make it unique among its kind.

Hepatitis is characterized by the presence in the blood of an antigen called HB-AG. This antigen turns up in different forms in different parts of the body, all of which can be measured to test the course of the disease. In studies, figuring the effect of a treatment against hepatitis becomes simple: measure the levels of antigen at various places and see which, if any, have gone down.

In the first interferon test with hepatitis, at Stanford, four patients with both hepatitis and chronic liver disease received daily interferon doses. It was found that interferon treatment seemed to have greater effects on some forms of the antigen than others. High enough doses over long enough periods of time, however, decreased all the various markers of the disease's activity. The study was hopeful but not conclusive.

A second test used fibroblast interferon in chimpanzees and indicated that interferon goes after the virus where it multiplies, not merely once it is loose in the system. And a third test, also with chimps, showed that an interferon inducer could also lower hepatitis indicators.

At Stanford, Drs. Merigan and William Robinson combined interferon with a long-standing chemical treatment that had had so-so success with hepatitis. They gave the dual treatment to some 200 patients with chronic hepatitis and all showed marked signs of improvement. Two responded with total elimination of active signs.

The interferon community was euphoric. Here was a case in which interferon could help wipe out a major health concern. It looked, for a time, as if it would be the protein's first point of impact with the world at large.

At nearly the same time as the interferon trials were showing positive results, a pair of virologists in New York were rounding up homosexuals to test a development of their own. They wanted gay men because their incidence of chronic hepatitis runs far above that of the general population. And the drug they wanted to test was a putative vaccine against the disease. Instead of going after the virus with dead viruses, as was traditional, the pair isolated an antigen from human blood that stimulated the immune system to attack the hepatitis. In the trials with 1083 homosexual volunteers, 96 percent were protected from the disease, a stunning achievement.

So, interferon was challenged and perhaps overwhelmed, as the best preventative of hepatitis. But what about treating those who already carry the disease? Vaccines cannot help in these cases.

Merigan has found that a combination of interferon with a drug called ara-A eliminated signs of chronic infection in 44 percent of patients in his study. These results were exciting enough to start him planning a full double-blind study of the treatment.

Eliminating the chronic-carrier-state of hepatitis is vitally important because this is how the disease spreads among humans. In the words of Dr. Robert M. Friedman: "This is the first time anybody has ever really achieved anything for the carrier state in chronic hepatitis, and it has the promise of being an effective therapy. Even if Dr. Merigan doesn't cure everybody, he's certainly cutting down on the infectivity of the patients."

The Common Cold. One of medicine's age-old pipe dreams is to find a cure for the common cold. Of course, the common cold isn't really a single disease, but a tangled web of variously related problems that generate the familiar symptoms of runny nose, watery eyes, and a generally lousy feeling. Interferon comes closer to being a genuine cold preventative than anything ever known, but it doesn't quite solve the problem.

In 1972, a test by the Medical Research Council of Great Britain determined quite soundly that interferon can take the sting out of colds. Massive doses of the protein given in thirty-nine doses over four days, reduced the symptoms and virus shedding of volunteers who had been exposed to a cold virus.

Throughout the field, interferon experts accept the facts shown in this study and others, that interferon treatments can be useful in preventing or moderating colds. But there's a catch.

In the experiments the volunteers were exposed to colds. The testers knew that colds were in the offing for the participants and that interferon treatment wouldn't have to go on too long. But in real life, who knows when one might catch cold? The only way to guard against ever getting a cold would be to take interferon treatments every day. The barriers to this aren't just interferon's overwhelming expense. As genetically engineered interferon hits the market, the cost will go down and interferon nasal sprays might become generally affordable. The bigger problem is whether a steady diet of interferon is a good idea.

The body eliminates interferon as quickly as it can once a virus has been quelled. Many researchers are convinced that nature doesn't do this without good reason. They figure that chronic, high levels of interferon may have deleterious effects on the body. Interferon's raw biological power makes it impossible for cells to function normally when it's around. In the face of a life-threatening virus infection or a potentially fatal cancer, the problems this altered state may bring are minor by comparison. But the built-up drawbacks of years of interferon therapy can easily outweigh the benefits from staving off a few days or weeks of stuffy noses.

So, the likelihood of seeing an interferon-based permanent anti-cold vaccine are slim. Still, perhaps greater understanding of how interferon works will make one possible in time.

This isn't to say that interferon won't play a hand in fighting colds. The scenario painted by scientists has interferon up on the drug store shelf next to *Dristan* and *Excedrin* as a medication you take at the first hints of a cold. Its effects, however, will be far greater than those of patent medicines. Unlike today's cold treatments, interferon won't just alleviate symptoms. Odds are that once a person begins taking interferon nose drops, the cold will be stopped, and will gradually fade away.

When used during the few days of a cold, interferon's effects on the body shouldn't be too serious, and the savings to society from workers with colds who will be able to stay on the job will be enormous.

Another potential use for interferon cold sprays is as a temporary cold preventative for people who want to make absolutely sure they don't get sick during a few specific days. A salesman, for instance, might want to start taking interferon a few days before major sales presentations; it will ensure that he won't get sniffles on the big day. An opera star might want to use interferon to guarantee a clear throat on performance night during a local cold epidemic. An executive who often gets colds when seasons change might use interferon to keep immune during that period in order not to lose valuable time at work. A couple on the eve of their long awaited vacation might want to make sure their trip is uninterrupted by a cold's symptoms.

All of these are temporary treatments. The interferon's effect will wear off about a day after the last application. In this way, interferon will perform as a vastly improved, more potent form of the cold medications we are familiar with today. In a few years you may hear a TV pitchman telling you to "Give your cold to Interferon."

Despite the fact that interferon's earliest known abilities were against viruses, and despite the positive results of many anti-viral interferon experiments, some voices in the field raise serious questions about what role the protein will eventually play in virus medication. They point to the recent development of the hepatitis vaccine as showing the real possibility that advances in other forms of virology will outstrip interferon in controlling viruses. If vaccines that stimulate the immune system become common, the need for a virus-controlling medicine will be virtually nil.

More ominously, they wonder about the relative value of interferon protection today against antibody protection tomorrow. Their disquiet stems from the fact that interferon only protects a recipient from viruses while it is elevated within the body. The minute interferon levels drop, the patient is every bit as vulnerable to a given virus as before treatment. Nature's system, however, doesn't pass away so thoughtlessly.

In the natural state, each virus infection that hits us creates the antibodies that will protect us from any future attack by that strain. As we come in contact with—and fight off—viruses we steadily become better protected against them. If we are always avoiding minor virus infections by using interferon, we won't ever build up those reserves of antibodies for future infections. We'll avoid the cold or flu today, but what will be the cost for tomorrow? Will we become especially vulnerable to a sort of super-flu, one not caught in time with a protective spray? Will it do more damage to our unprotected systems than a lifetime of ordinary infections? No one is certain, but the possibility can't be discounted.

Dr. Derek Burke sums up the negative position cogently: "When interferon was discovered we had very few anti-viral drugs. We still have only a relative few. But recently we have gone from a profound pessimism about synthetic virus treatments to a solid optimism. I think synthetics will be the drugs of choice in many virus conditions. And I don't think I'll see a broad spectrum cold treatment that really works in my lifetime.

"I think all we can hope to do is to live with the common cold and flu and the mumps, use vaccines where they're appropriate and save interferon for the limited number of life-threatening viruses where synthetics aren't available or don't work."

Many others in the field, it should be made clear, see the situation much more positively. They believe that once interferon is cheap and widely available, it will become as common a treatment as any well-known drug of the moment. They feel that fears about antibodies are overstated, and the effectiveness of the drug is such that it will surpass the expectations of overly cautious practitioners.

Still, the negative scenario raises the ironic possibility that interferon will be shut out in the field that gave it birth, and will stand or fall on its abilities against cancers and other non-virus ills originally considered irrelevant to its existence.

chapter 4

THE WONDER DRUG POTENTIAL

4

A drug that made it possible for doctors to transplant organs safely, without fear of infection or rejection, would be considered a masterful medical development. Experiments that could help unlock the secrets behind Down's Syndrome, a congenital condition that produces malformed, retarded babies, would be hailed as a significant step forward in knowledge. A substance that attacked vicious parasites that bring blight and blindness to the people of the underdeveloped nations would excite researchers everywhere. A protein that guarded plants from many of their most destructive diseases would mean vast savings for farmers and expansion of the world's precious food supply.

Each of these potentials would be remarkable. Interferon has them all. So widespread have interferon's abilities become—so far beyond the standard potencies against cancer and viruses—that the protein has taken on a character of virtual omniscience in treatment. There seems to be no body system where interferon doesn't have some impact. There seem to be few conditions that the protein leaves entirely untouched.

Such all-embracing powers are unheard-of in medicine. Many scientists have grown deeply skeptical about interferon simply because so many totally different abilities have been attributed to it. Nothing, they feel, can do all these things, and the plethora of claims must be a smoke screen to obscure the insufficiencies of interferon's performance in viral and cancer tests. Interferon surely would have been more readily accepted by the scientific community if its properties weren't so totally out-of-line with all that has come before.

But these abilities aren't the specious powers of a fad cure; they arise from sober scientific studies. And while some of them will almost certainly not come to fruition, others almost certainly will. Interferon is simply the most versatile potential medication to have been seen in many decades, perhaps ever.

The extent of interferon's ancillary abilities has grown as research has expanded beyond answering the basic question of what it is and how it works. Some capabilities arise as logical offshoots of experimentation in other areas. Others are indications from preliminary lab studies with animals.

Some of interferon's side benefits seem to grow out of its ability simply to make the cell stronger. A cell that is primed to overcome the massive invasion of a virus will also, unintentionally, be in excellent shape to repel less potent attackers. Other interferon possibilities derive from the protein's intimate relationship with the body's immune system.

When first discovered, interferon was thought to be more or less a Lone Ranger, riding through the body and warning against the approach of viruses. But as study has continued and more information accumulated, the reality has turned out to be more complex than first imagined. Interferon was discovered to be not a single substance but a family, and today most experts speak of an interferon system encompassing a variety of responses by different types of cells to different situations. The interferon protein itself is merely one key element in this system, which touches most aspects of cell activity and immune system responses. Responses by this larger interferon system, rather than the direct anti-viral properties of the protein, help explain some of the additional potentialities of the drug.

All these capabilities, you should remember, are highly speculative. Many are derived from solitary studies or even by extrapolation from studies on different topics. Consider the incredible supply squeeze in crucial virus and cancer experiments, and you can imagine the difficulty at getting enough interferon to study purported side abilities.

As interferon had to wait for virology to catch up with it, these capabilities will have to wait for interferon research to catch up with them. Questions about viruses and cancer must be answered first, before the side issues can be addressed. Until then, these interferon traits range from probable to unlikely potentials that have yet to be established by hard scientific evidence.

Clearly, the most important of interferon's additional talents centers on its modulation of the body's immune system. The flexible protein can either increase or suppress immune effects, depending upon when and how it is given. Increased immune response will help cancer patients by increasing their chance of fighting off infections.

Decreased immune response will help both cancer patients and others by making organ transplants less dangerous and more likely to succeed.

Building immune response will lessen one of the worst long-term side effects of cancer chemotherapy and radiation treatments, namely the wearing away of the body's ability to stave off infections of all sorts. The volatile cells of the immune system are killed along with cancer cells, leaving the patient essentially defenseless against all the germs and viruses and fungi around him.

Interferon therapy, apart from any action it has against tumors, seems to stimulate the recipient's immune system. This raises the possibility that interferon could be used to help patients stay free from infection while under treatment. It also carries some hope for those born with defective immune systems. Dampening immune response, on the other hand, could lead to more successful and less difficult operations in the near future.

When an organ is transplanted from one person to another, the recipient's body will attack and destroy it. The immune system will see the alien organ as a massive invasion, an infection, and do everything possible to get rid of it. Thus, the matching of minute details between transplant organs and recipients is so important to doctors. It is why kidney transplants should be between immediate blood relatives, particularly siblings, whose bodies will be most like each other.

Even with the most careful matching imagineable, however, the recipient's immune system still has a good chance of sensing the differences and attacking the new organ. The only way doctors have been able to cope with this touchy situation is to use chemicals and radiation to shock the recipient's immune system into total inactivity before, during, and for a good while after a transplant operation.

The stultified immune system can't reject the new organ, but in the meantime the patient is totally exposed to infection or disease. On top of that, the immuno-suppressing techniques carry with them severe side effects. This is one of those cases in modern medicine where the cure is almost as bad as the problem.

Interferon appears to handle this role better than existing treatments. When interferon is administered very early in an immune response, it dampens the functioning of the immune system. This dampening effect can be maintained for long periods without any apparent lasting destructive effect. So, interferon could conceivably keep a transplant recipient's immune system in check while the body gets used to the presence of a new organ.

The greatest advantage, though, is that instead of leaving the immuno-suppressed patient vulnerable to virus infections, interferon will simultaneously make one impervious to them. In many transplant cases, viruses kill the patient before the transplanted organ can even begin to function. In cases of kidney transplants, virtually 100 percent of patients have to survive both the operation, the immune response, and virus infections before they are out of the woods. Interferon immuno-suppression would largely alleviate two of these problems.

Part of the evidence for this ability comes from interferon mouse studies. Mice that received kidney transplants quickly developed a kind of virus, called Type C, that led to virus-based tumors. Normal immuno-suppressive techniques don't eliminate the Type C cells; in fact, there was some indication they may have helped stimulate them. Interferon therapy, on the other hand, wiped out Type C cells in some animals and reduced levels in others. None of the mice who received interferon developed tumors. As a report on the immune properties of interferon stated: "Interferons appear to be almost ideally suited to the needs of transplantation medicine because they may achieve immunosuppression in the body together with resistance to viruses and possibly other intracellular parasites." Double-blind, placebo-controlled studies of interferon's effects on human kidney transplant patients are underway at two clinics.

Deeply fascinating but of less imminent importance and of possibly tremendous long-range value is the strange link that has been uncovered between interferon and Down's Syndrome, the cause of the retardation condition known as mongoloidism. Victims are born with an extra chromosome which leaves them with slanted eyes, stunted minds, and shortened life spans.

On the surface, it would seem that interferon and mental retardation couldn't have less to do with one another. But consider an interesting coincidence in nature: The genetic information that causes cells to respond to the presence of interferon is on chromosome 21. The chomosomal anomaly behind Down's Syndrome is an extra copy of chromosomal 21.

Study of this relationship has been performed by Lois and Charles Epstein, a husband and wife team from the University of California at San Francisco. Children with Down's Syndrome are known to have immunological problems; they are usually prone to infection and have a higher-than-average chance of developing leukemia—but no one knows why. The Epsteins found a clue. Cells from children with Down's Syndrome, they found, are especially sensitive to interferon, and this heightened sensitivity may disrupt their immune system response.

"I am interested in interferon and my husband is interested in genetics," says Lois Epstein, "and we used both of our backgrounds to pull these two things together." The researchers knew that the gene coding for interferon sensitivity is on chromosome 21—the same chromosome that causes Down's Syndrome when an extra copy is present. But human genes are sometimes difficult to study experimentally. To understand the exact chemical nature of the interferon response, the researchers turned to laboratory mice.

Working with postdoctoral fellow David Cox, the Epsteins managed to identify the mouse chromosome—number 16—that determines interferon response in mice.[1]

The discovery opened an exciting possibility. The UCSF scientists reasoned that the chromosome segment responsible for Down's Syndrome and the gene for the interferon response might be linked in mice, as they are in people. Using sophisticated embryological techniques, the Epsteins have been trying to breed mouse embryos that have an extra chromosome 16 to see if the animals would develop a syndrome resembling the human disease that results from an extra chromosome 21. They hope this research will produce the first mouse model for Down's Syndrome.

"We now have made mouse embryos with an extra chromosome 16," says Lois Epstein. "They look grossly different from normal mouse embryos. They have swollen bodies. They have congenital abnormalities of the heart which is also true of patients with Down's Syndrome, although the defects are not exactly the same."

One research difficulty, explains Lois Epstein, is that these mouse embryos, with an extra chomosome 16, ordinarily do not survive to a live birth. In order to prolong the growing but defective embryos, the Epsteins are in the process of breeding mouse chimeras. A chimera is an animal with a mixture of parents. In this case, the chimeras will be the offspring of four parents. The scientists fuse two embryos—one with cells from normal parents and one with cells that have extra copies of chromosome 16—obtained by mating a normal animal with an experimental one that carries chromosomes rearranged by the scientists.

This new breed of experimental mice should give researchers a better understanding of a serious and common form of mental retardation. The research project has come full circle. Cells from patients with Down's Syndrome originally helped scientists begin to explain how interferon acts on cells. Now basic research on interferon may help victims of that genetic disease.

Interferon research may also bring aid and comfort to victims of another seemingly unrelated problem—obesity. In what may be the single most creative use of interferon in an experiment, a pair of researchers at the Medical College of Wisconsin in Milwaukee tested the protein's ability to slow the breakdown of fibroblast (muscle) tissue into fat.

As people grow older, their muscle tissue gradually gives way to fat cells. Any cellulite-hater or jowl-jiggler can attest to that. In the Wisconsin study, scientists Susan Keay and Sidney Grossberg exposed to interferon mouse muscle cells that predictably break down into fat. They found that "interferon can inhibit the expression of the change in genetic program involving conversion of one cell type into another." In other words, the protein slowed the shift from muscle to fat in the mouse systems.[2]

What does this mean for people? According to the testers, "it is tempting to speculate that the conversion of (muscle tissue) into (fat) . . . manifested in aging or obesity might be affected by interferon."

One can imagine treatments of interferon for the chronically obese, whose bodies convert food into fat so fast they endanger themselves. By slowing this destructive cycle, interferon could increase one's lifespan and enjoyment remarkably.

If the protein's side effects don't prove too bothersome, interferon might also be used in middle age as a means of warding off the fat shift that marks our movement into the golden years. It could, literally, help keep us younger longer.

In some underdeveloped parts of the world, however, longer and more beautiful life is a meaningless concept. In addition to the viruses that plague us, people from underdeveloped nations face malnutrition and other scourges of poverty, and they are afflicted by parasitic diseases that blind, maim, and kill.

Trachoma, an eye infection that strikes 500 million people a year and is the world's leading cause of blindness, is one such disease. It is caused by a family of parasites named Chlamydiae. The milder eye inflammation, conjunctivitis, also stems from this destructive clan.

Interferon can handle parasites like this. The reason seems to be that some parasite infections resemble viruses. They contain DNA and RNA genetic coding, and go through a dormant phase that is similar to a virus' eclipse stages, which occurs shortly after it begins to spread in a system.

In the lab, it has been shown that the Chlamydiae agents can induce interferon production in cells, much as a virus would. And parasite growth is slowed in both cells and eggs when interferon is present. The only attempt at treating an animal suffering from trachoma with interferon failed, but the dosage was so unbelievably low—thirty-two units as compared to a typical dose of three million units—that the failure means little.

Barring decent tests in animals and humans, it can't be said that interferon will help alleviate these problems; but the suggestion that it might registers strongly with some scientists.

Interferon's response to some other parasites is far more complex. Protozoan parasites, for instance, which are responsible for malaria, Chagas' disease, and many other devastating conditions, only seem responsive to interferon once they have settled within the confine of a cell. In the lab, they are resistant.

Take, for example, the case of Plasmodium berghei, a malaria parasite. When mice were given injections of sporozoites—the raw stuff that mosquitoes manufacture to transmit malaria—to stimulate P. berghei infection, interferon showed peculiar potency. The sporozoites settle in the liver cells of their host where they shift into their active mode and marshal forces for an attack on the red blood cells. In the liver cells, interferon and chemicals which induce interferon production all showed enormous effectiveness. When the infection reached the red blood cells, however, effectiveness dropped off to near zero.

In the case of another parasite, trypanosomes, one set of results shows that interferon reduces the parasitic burden in mouse livers, while another shows that it increases the degree of activity.

One disease reaction in particular which could alleviate many worries and fretting in rural America involves ticks. These fat pests inflict quite a few people each summer with Rocky Mountain spotted fever, sometimes with serious consequences, even death. Interferon appears to stop the development of Rocky Mountain spotted fever.

While some of these results are encouraging, the scientific evidence on interferon's parasitic talents is as yet unavailable. A study concluded: "The mechanism of the antiparasitic effects reported is at present unknown, although it seems clear that it is mediated by cells, as is the antiviral effect."[3]

Interferon may also provide an effective treatment or screening substance for some of the most mysterious chronic diseases known, the slow viruses. When a person becomes senile prematurely, it is probably a slow virus—the Creutzfeld-Jacob syndrome. A victim of multiple sclerosis also suffers from slow virus effects. Amyotrophic lateral sclerosis, the illness that sapped the strength and then the life of Lou Gehrig, probably comes from a similar source. Even arthritis may be tied to slow viruses.

Slow virus is most likely not a substance, but an effect. Many neurological problems are thought to derive from low-level viral activity that lingers in the body for years before manifesting itself as illness. The amounts of virus in the body are so low they don't set off our immune system alarms or make us immediately "ill." The disease that results after years of exposure grows from gentle, persistent irritation of nerves, muscles, or brain cells.

Although these conditions are incurable today, preliminary interferon indications hold the hope that the coming generation may be spared the lingering death of slow viruses. The link between "slow virus" diseases and interferon is fairly obvious. If interferon works against viruses, and other infections that act like viruses, why not against slow virus, too?

Unfortunately, there have been no significant human tests with any of these conditions. But a suggestive piece of work has been done in lab studies at Albert Einstein Medical Center in New York. There, researchers found that if you take cells—any cells from a patient with multiple sclerosis—and infect them with a virus, they respond normally by putting out interferon, like all normal cells. But if you infect them with measles virus, they don't respond. This is a strong reason to implicate measles virus in the disease, as if the bodies of these people are incapable of defending themselves against this particular affliction.

M.S., then, may arise after years of irritation within the body by a measles virus that the body is powerless to protect against. The amount of virus in the system remains quite low, so the immune system never comes into play. And, irregularities in the system somehow make it impossible for interferon to recognize the virus for what it is. After years and years of slow viral action, effects begin to appear. These effects we call multiple sclerosis.

None of this, of course, is proved; it's all speculation upon fascinating, but rather shaky evidence. Still, Mathilde Krim feels the indications make creating a mental picture worthy:

"All we have in this field are hunches. We think they may be caused by viruses or slow viruses and interferon would certainly be active against these. But at what stage? Perhaps by the time symptoms appear, it's too late for interferon to do anything.

"I can envision a scenario in which interferon is used as a test rather than as a treatment for, say M.S. It would be possible to test babies—although only those from families with a predisposition toward the disease or who show some other early sign of trouble—with interferon, just as we now do with several other early tests.

"The interferon test would involve taking a little blood and exposing cells to measles virus. If they produce interferon, we know the child won't develop the disease later in life. But if they fail to produce interferon, we know the child is a potential victim. We can put him on interferon therapy, just like we put diabetics on insulin therapy. We could prevent the possibility of the condition occurring from birth."

So incredible is the expanse of interferon's potential that it doesn't stop with animal diseases. Plants, too, apparently protect themselves with a protein related to interferon.

Israeli virologists have been making jokes lately about how *their* interferon grows on trees. They have a right to laugh because an Israeli scientist actually has found a substance that looks like interferon, acts like interferon, that probably is interferon—except it's produced by plant cells, rather than animal ones.

Dr. Ilan Sela of Hebrew University in Jerusalem discovered the anti-viral factor in tobacco plants. It is responsible for the plants' resistance to disease in a manner similar to interferon with animals. Botanists pinpointed this resistance artificially by adding a special gene, called the N-gene, into the genetic material.

At a 1980 symposium, Sela explained that the plant factor and animal interferon are alike in several ways. Their structures, reactions to acids, and other basic components seem identical. And, like interferon, the plant factor is produced only after a plant containing the N-gene has been infected with a virus. Only a tiny amount of the material—four or five molecules per cell—is required for viral resistance against a wide range of invaders.

The plant factor even demonstrates the same type of enzymatic activity as interferon; it induces an enzyme that snips messenger-RNA molecules. The manner of regulation in the cell also approximates that of interferon.

Plant interferon, Sela believes, could bring about a revolution in world agriculture: virus-free plants. The importance of such highly resistant strains to a world struggling to feed itself is incalculable.

Sela also holds hope of using plants as factories to produce an anti-viral protein that will work in humans. The plant cells generate far more of their N-gene molecules than an animal cell does interferon. So far, though, Sela has been unable to get his plant protein to intervene reliably in animal infections. The search for a vegetable protein that also works in humans should proceed apace the race to produce genetically engineered interferon.

What interferon does to cells, whether in the case of viruses, cancers, or other diseases, is the primary interest of scientists in the field. But the question most often asked by curious non-scientists is: What does it do to people? How do interferon recipients feel?

The protein's effects aren't limited to cell activity. It will be used as a medication in people who have hearts, minds, and feelings. The personal impact of interferon remains every bit as important to explore as its medical prowess.

chapter 5

THE CHOSEN FEW

5

Twice each week, Peter DeFilippo rides a bus from his central New Jersey home to Manhattan's Memorial Sloan-Kettering Cancer Center. Upstairs, a technician gives him a shot of a liquid that looks much like watered-down apple juice. While he's rolling down his sleeves, she prepares an ice chest with enough filled hypodermic needles to hold him until his next visit. DeFilippo, a burly, balding, former Air Force Captain, grabs his chilly parcel and heads back home.

Peter DeFilippo has cancer and his treatment is interferon. About three years ago he went to the doctor because a small, dark mole beneath his ear had been acting up. The diagnosis was melanoma, a potentially fatal skin cancer.

After the discovery, DeFilippo's existence took a sharp downward turn. He went under the knife twice. Doctors blasted him with experimental fast-neutron radiation therapy. They injected him with two kinds of chemotherapy agents. Both made him violently ill. And after all the treatments, his cancer came back.

"I had been reading about interferon," he recalls, "and I thought, I need a miracle or something because regular therapy's not going to help me."

He also wanted a better quality of life. "I don't want to jam life in to make up for lost time. I just want to preserve the quality of my life for the time I have left. I don't want to get up every day and throw up."[1]

DeFilippo is one of just 150 or so cancer victims to receive interferon in the United States. He is among the chosen because he is lucky and because he refuses to give up. Over his years of treatment, he says, he wandered "from doctor to hospital to hospital to doctor, and as soon as this ends, if I continue to have spread, I'll be back on the treadmill again."

When treatments began to fail, DeFilippo dragged himself to

countless specialists, read everything he could find on new treatments for his disorder, even presented his doctor with a list of phone numbers for specialists in experimental treatments. When Sloan-Kettering put out the call, he was there.

But even with all his exertions, the plucky ex-fly jockey would never have gotten his first drop of interferon if he hadn't fulfilled a broad range of detailed research criteria: He was healthy, except for the cancer. He had taken all available accepted treatments. He had the right kind of cancer at the right stage of development. He could get to the hospital easily. He had the right medical history and family background.

Sloan-Kettering doctors drummed into his head the fact that he was part of an experiment; he was not receiving a course of treatment in the regular sense. No one held out any promise of improvement. He shouldn't raise his hopes. All doctors would state was that the treatment probably wouldn't make him any worse.

Still, he said, "I'm hopeful. The chemotherapy didn't seem to work, and I had to do something different if I was going to survive. This looked like the most hopeful thing to do."

To keep in shape and keep his spirits up, DeFilippo stretches and runs twenty-five miles each week. "I'm afraid to stop, to be honest with you," he admits. "I think as long as I can do these things, I am healthy and it can't spread. Of course, I don't know whether that's true or not."

Fortunately, he hasn't suffered the chills and fatigue that have occasionally struck others in his test group. So, each day, apparently in perfect health except for a slash of scar tissue on his neck from the treatments, he jogs across the Jersey plateau. And twice each week he rides the smelly bus into Manhattan for his dose. And he hopes.

Today's interferon recipients are a small band of hardy cancer veterans. They have run the gamut of treatments and have the scars and horror stories to show for it. They have reached a place beyond reasonable hope where only sheer determination keeps them on the lookout for any new treatment that might improve their odds. But even while they are looking, they sense deep down that their cancer will eventually win. No matter how good an experimental treatment they find, they sense that the real benefits will come for those who follow. Not for them.

Interferon for most of them comes after a long hard trip through surgery, chemotherapy, radiation, and far more exotic treatments. They may have given up on their individual chance to beat cancer—most seem to believe that the best possible goal is to hold off the inevitable, not defeat it—but they still feel a deep hope, a deep need to hope, that others will be served by their suffering. Interferon is their chance to give something to the world through a disease that has struck them irrationaly and mercilessly.

"It's a good feeling," says interferon recipient Helen De Rise. "It makes you feel like what you've gone through may be of value to someone later on."

To some extent, today's interferon recipients are where they are through happenstance. Edward Tyler, a patient in Gutterman's test in Houston says, "I was simply fortunate enough to have been here at just the time that the money came through from the Cancer Society. It allowed them to buy enough interferon to test people like me. Right place, right time."

Despite Peter DeFilippo's pluck, he would not have become an interferon recipient had he not been fortunate enough to live close to a major cancer center. Today's studies of interferon as an anticancer agent are centered in ten of these huge treatment and research facilities. They have the only supplies of the scarce medication, and they dole it out under rigid controls.

The ten institutions chosen for the initial cancer studies with interferon are: M.D. Anderson Hospital and Tumor Institute, Houston; Memorial Sloan-Kettering Institute for Cancer Research, New York; Stanford University Medical Center, Palo Alto, California; Roswell Park Memorial Institute, Buffalo, New York; Columbia Uniersity College of Physicians and Surgeons, New York; UCLA Medical Center, Los Angeles; Yale University Medical Center, New Haven, Connecticut; University of Wisconsin Hospital, Madison; and Mount Sinai Medical Center, New York.

Since experimentation at all these large hospitals would utilize only 150 cancer victims, each center had enough suitable recipients on hand for the tests. When the deluge of requests, demands, pleas, and threats for receiving interferon came down, it was a sad fact that virtually no open places existed in any of the studies.

Those patients who did get in all followed a fairly similar course. They lived close to, or were patients at, one of the big institutions at the time the tests got underway. Either they or their personal physician knew about the tests and put their case before the researchers. And, most importantly, they fit the criteria.

In Edward Tyler's case, he asked his doctor at the Scot-White Clinic in Temple, Texas whether interferon would be of any use to him. Tyler had known of his cancer since 1975 when he had noticed a slight tinge of blood in his stool during a business trip to California. Surgery for rectal cancer followed. The doctors felt hopeful that they'd gotten it all. But months later, during a routine follow-up, they found a depressing metastasis, an inoperable tumor hugging the pelvis. Intensive radiation and chemotherapy ensued, and Tyler's tumor stabilized. But it hadn't gone away.

It was at this point that Tyler thought about interferon. He was in excellent health except for the looming background of his tumor. All the available treatments had been tried and he still had cancer. How could interferon hurt?

The doctors at Scot-White agreed and called Gutterman in Houston. The combination of a cancer that resisted treatment in a perfectly healthy person suited their needs and Tyler was called to M.D. Anderson for tests and interviews. After looking him over the testers agreed. He made a good candidate. He was admitted to the program.

HOW ONE IS CHOSEN

How do scientists select the patients who enter the exclusive fraternity of interferon recipients? Their decisions are based on precise guidelines that derive from the requirements of producing scientifically useful, reliable results. Despite their desire to help patients and cure people, their primary thought in setting up a human trial is gleaning important information. With interferon, these considerations are enormously intensified by the severe lack of supply.

With an ordinary drug, the progress of testing goes rather smoothly along a well-established, predictable course. In the beginning, a drug company or an independent researcher comes up with an idea, or a glimmering of experimental evidence, that holds some promise for development of a drug. The discoverers will gather money through grants or corporate backing to get a supply of material for testing. They will test for toxicity—the level at which the drug becomes lethal. They will give the drug to experimental animals at varying doses and in different manners, looking to see how the best effect is achieved. Then the researchers will move onto small human clinical trials. And, based upon those results, they may scale up to large human trials.

At each step, the experiments are designed entirely with the intention of yielding enough information to determine whether the move to the next step is justified. Whenever a drug fails to produce strong enough results, it is dropped. Only the best make it through the entire winnowing process to reach full-scale human trials, and only a few of those go on to become common medical tools.

With interferon, however, the system is stretched past its limit. Until very recently, there simply wasn't any supply of interferon to speak of. Now the supply exists, but it is so costly and so thinly spread among researchers that no individual has enough to mount even a large first-step toxicity test, let alone anything grander. Interferon is so dear, the thought of pumping enough of it into test subjects to show toxicity makes researchers pale. As for widespread human tests, they are impossible. There simply isn't enough interferon—anywhere—to perform them.

The supply situation has begun to ease, and the recent arrival of genetically engineered interferon will soon make the shortage a matter of history. But until now, interferon has never been plentiful enough to perform adequate tests at any level of development to produce a clear-cut picture of what is going on. Each step has been suggestive enough that someone has taken the risk to go further, but the normal scientific evidence for the move has never been possible to amass.

At each stage interferon has been a gamble. So far the gamble has paid off. But it's still like betting without a system. You can never be totally sure of what the next roll of the dice will bring.

Under the best of conditions, the movement through the labyrinth of testing goes in tiny steps. Each test either proves one small fact or eliminates it. The great mass of fact—like the points of color in a pointillist painting—creates the overall image of the drug's performance and usefulness.

With interferon, the steps have been even smaller than normal because the tests have been smaller. The smaller a test is, the more limited the conclusions that can be drawn from it. If you test one person, all you can say is that the drug cured one person. If you test half the people with a disease and all are cured, you can surmise that the drug is fairly effective, but not totally so. If you test many different patients under a range of circumstances, and all of your results follow your model for the drug's behavior, then you can tell with reasonable certainty what you have and how it works.

Right now there is no model for interferon's behavior and too small a supply to perform the wide ranging tests that would generate one. Interferon lies between the one-person test and the half-the-cases test. It falls in the realm of indications rather than facts. Five patients here, ten there, two or three somewhere else. It's exciting, enticing, and sometimes even disappointing, but there is never any conclusive information.

Because the number of tests and the number of recipients are limited, the design of the tests and the informational worthiness of the subjects become infintely important. With a normal drug, failed tests can be as valuable as those that work. A failure shows you where the boundary lies. Sometimes tests are designed to fail so that researchers can help fill in the all-important model of the drug's behavior. A drug that doesn't fail when it's supposed to, is as big a problem as one that doesn't work when it's supposed to.

But with interferon, failure, even now, could be fatal. If any among the few interferon tests fails to show some activity, the bad publicity could sink the entire field of inquiry. No researcher can fall back on the thought that somewhere in the horde of fellow scientists, someone will be getting positive results to offset it. Interferon testing is too small a field for that.

So interferon tests are designed to get positive responses. This is done by focusing work on cancers that have shown some inclination toward interferon response in the past. The first interferon work in humans, quite casually, involved a bone cancer called osteogenic sarcoma. Interferon seemed to cause a response, so osteogenic sarcoma had an inside track for future interferon work. Other inconclusive evidence—called anecdotal evidence among scientists—touched a few other cancers. These few cancers form the backbone of interferon testing today. They are included not because they are worse than other cancers, nor because their victims suffer more from them. The simple fact is that researchers feel that these particular ailments offer the best chance today for positive results.

A second group of cancers makes it into the tests because they strike very often and resist existing treatments rather well. Scientists place these cancers in tests for two reasons. Since they are common, they provide a wide population of potential test subjects allowing the researcher to be choosy, to get the cleanest results. Also, because of their commonness, any success will have maximum positive impact, both in terms of helping patients and directing attention and money into the field.

The third group considered for testing includes cancers of particular ease or value in the lab. Myeloma, for instance, a bone cancer, secretes an identifiable protein into the blood. As the tumors get bigger, the amount of protein increases. As they shrink, it decreases. So, measuring drug effects on myeloma tumors can be rather exact, enabling researchers much greater accuracy.

Once the cancers to be tested are chosen, researchers have to determine the best kind of patients to test. They want all those tested to be as much alike as possible for the obvious reason that the fewer differences between the patients the more consistent and reliable results should be. They may want to eliminate certain types of people outright—some ethnic groups, for instance, may have much worse recovery rates for a cancer than the normal population, which could distort the test results.

They want cancers at a particular stage of development. In early tests, this is usually after every existing treatment has been tried and failed. For instance, patients still may have breast cancer that surgery and radiotherapy have failed to eradicate. Or myeloma that has not responded to several other treatments. Earlier treatments could conceivably affect the way a subject responds to what is being tested, so similarity of treatment is important.

The rules for selecting the disease and subjects for a study are called protocols. They are adhered to so strictly, it prompted one researcher to exclaim that "the sad and brutal fact is that if my own mother didn't meet the protocol she could not get interferon today."

GETTING IN: A GAMBLE

In some cases, a cancer victim's desperate search for interferon can become a genuine tragedy. Hundreds have expended the precious time cancer allowed them in vain attempts to secure the drug. In mid-1980, the *Wall Street Journal* reported the case of a pseudonymous cancer victim named Mary Malone. That spring, she had seen an erroneous press release that announced interferon sales to private doctors by a Florida company, Life Sciences, Inc. At that point, Mary, a thirty-seven year old Florida dental assistant, had undergone a long round of chemotherapy for breast cancer that had left her "weak and sick all the time," and hadn't stopped the spread of the disease. After rejecting an even stronger dose of anti-cancer chemicals—because "my body just can't take any more"—Mary was receiving experimental immune system therapy using tuberculosis bacteria that gave her a wracking cough, when she heard about the false interferon sales.[2]

She, along with hundreds of others, called Maxwell Powell, Life Sciences' co-founder and director, and left him feeling low. "She has nowhere to go. It's very depressing. If I'd had some in my desk drawer when that lady called I'd have given it to her."

But he didn't, so Mary went on a cross-country trek for someone willing to treat her with the drug she hoped could stop her cancer and free her from the draining side effects of other treatments she'd tried. "I have nothing to lose," she said, "Maybe it'll help. At least it isn't a poison."

But the odds were stacked against her. And she couldn't beat them. She went to Houston, where doctors told her more chemotherapy and possibly more surgery would have to be tried before they could put her at the bottom of their 100-person waiting list. She travelled to Buffalo, but the Roswell Park Memorial Institute staffers said they couldn't accept anyone who had already received chemotherapy. Her travel and phone bills mounted, and so did her rejections. Five interferon testing institutions turned her down.

"Maybe if I were the Shah's daughter," she said bitterly, "I'd have better luck."

The viewpoints of researcher and patients—in fact, even those of the researcher and his own values and personality—differ when confronted by deserving people who cry for interferon. The patient wants to survive at any cost. The researcher wants to learn at any ethical price. The human side of the tester wants to save people because they are good or worthy or young. But the cold, calculating side must win out; pure informational needs must prevail if we are ever to determine how a new substance works and who it will help best. It is a necessary sacrifice for all concerned. The lucky ones aren't necessarily those who receive interferon. The truly lucky ones will be the next generation who will reap the benefits gained by today's work and sacrifices.

Mary Malone's despair about not receiving interferon points up the greater tragedy beyond her personal disappointment: even if she'd gotten it, she might not have been helped. "People don't understand," says Thomas L. Dao of Roswell Park, "not only the scarcity (of interferon) but that we still don't know how good it is."

"There is still no assurance," argues Dr. Norman Chirigos of the National Cancer Institute, "that any cancer patient will respond to interferon."

Thousands of cancer victims see interferon as a remedy; they see the institutions that have interferon supplies as places of treatment. But the institutions are not working to save a patient. They aren't aiming to cure anyone in particular. They aren't using their interferon to save a life.

They are trying to learn. Their research is directed to the long-term control of cancer.

Cancer patients who are turned down for interferon trials—and 99 percent are automatically eliminated by sheer scarcity—aren't less lucky than those who get in. The interferon volunteer is accepting an absolute blind shot, while the refused patient will receive treatment that science knows, without question, has some level of effectiveness.

The risk in the interferon trial isn't that interferon does nothing, but that we don't know yet exactly how it does what it does, how strongly it works, what affects its performance, what personal factors might be involved, how high the dose should be, and a host of seminal questions.

Inductees into interferon trials today are literally human guinea pigs who are willing to let their bodies be used as study mediums in which scientists can try to answer these questions. Only when the questions are answered can genuine treatment begin.

Helen De Rise realized full well that interferon was experimental when she became involved with it, but she had little to lose from trying it. She had struggled for seven years against multiple melanoma, a cancer that usually dispatches its victims swiftly. But something in De Rise's makeup slowed the cancer's spread. Still, its toll on her had been numerous, painful surgeries and bouts with chemotherapy, pills, radiation, everything.

It had begun with a mole on her ankle. She first noticed it when in her early twenties. And she would forget about it except when it was skinned or bumped against her bicycle chain. When she was twenty-eight, she noticed it had turned black and bled at a touch. She went to her dermatologist who knew in a single look that she had melanoma.

"For years," she recalls, "the treatments were able to cap the cancer. It kept spreading but each round of treatment would hold it at that position. By this spring it had reached most of my lymph system, but no vital organs. Then it overran the normal treatments. It began to spread."

She talked to her doctor at Mt. Sinai Medical Center in New York about interferon. It was not the first experimental possibility they had discussed. Whenever she heard of something new she'd ask him about it.

With interferon, he decided following up was a good idea and he set about getting De Rise into a treatment program somewhere. At first it looked as though she was headed for Roswell Park in Buffalo, but that fell through. Then Dr. Susan Krown at Sloan-Kettering answered their call.

Because she had one of the chosen cancers and had withstood all previous treatment without losing her general health, De Rise was considered a solid candidate for testing dosage levels. Her treatments might or might not have any permanent positive effect on her cancer, but they would put her illness to use for the future and she liked that thought.

Dr. Rauscher sums up the gamble of interferon testing today rather neatly: "Today some 40 to 50 percent of patients in the tests are responding. This also means that 50 to 60 percent are not responding at all." These percentages may improve as more is known about interferon and its relationship to cancer; but there's no guarantee of that and no guarantee for today's recipients of any help at all.

As hard a fact as it may be to accept, the truth is that interferon studies are—and must be—set up as they are for reasons that have nothing to do with cancer patients. The cancer patient is like a donor in these experiments; he is giving his body to the researcher to test ideas or assumptions the scientist has. The researcher's primary interest in the study must lie with confirming or refuting the assumption or hypothesis being tested. These assumptions are specific and constructed to garner the most helpful scientific evidence, rather than to produce the best situation for the patient.

For example, at Roswell Park Memorial Institute, Dr. William A. Carter is giving interferon to about thirty patients with breast cancer, melanoma, bladder cancer, or prostate cancer. The question he is trying to answer, though, isn't whether interferon cures these cancers. He wants to know whether fibroblast interferon, which comes from muscle cells, shows a better or different anti-tumor response than leukocyte interferon, which comes from white blood cells. So, his patients are split between the two types of interferon and he compares their reactions.

At M. D. Anderson, Dr. Jordan Gutterman is adding interferon to the mix of treatments used against breast cancer. Does interferon, added to the array, produce any improvement in survival? Other tests are designed to see if interferon shows any activity at all in patients who have not responded to accepted treatments. And there are further tests to determine whether certain people have a more pronounced reaction to interferon therapy than others.

Such scientific questions stand behind the selection of patients for these studies and the way they are set up. Because researchers know so little about interferon, the structure of the studies has purposefully been made highly varied. Some of the studies use low dosages for periods up to eighteen months. Others try high dosages for as little as six weeks. In some studies patients who don't show immediate response will be dropped right away, while in others they will be maintained to see if a long-term effect comes into play.

This variety, too, is part of the attempt to glean as much scientific knowledge as possible from the tests. When a patient enters an interferon program, he doesn't simply "get" interferon. He receives a certain amount of interferon, given in a certain manner for a prescribed length of time. The specific pattern of treatment might not be the one the doctor would choose to benefit that individual patient, but it's the best one for finding the answers the researcher needs.

In the discovery phase through which interferon is now passing, it's only good fortune when a cancer patient ends up with the program that will give the right dosage for the right length of time in the right way.

In such a circumstance, the patient's good luck could teach scientists a lot, but that's all it would be—luck. These tests are designed to help scientists learn enough so that the next round of tests can be more informed, and eventually knowledge can reach the point where the patient's receiving the right amounts and regimen of interferon is no longer a matter of guesswork, but of solid medical understanding.

HOW THE PROGRAMS ARE RUN

In America, interferon testing has been broad, but not particularly deep. Studies have looked at how interferon affects patients who receive it, but they have, by and large, lacked what scientists call controls—an equal and opposing group of patients who get nothing or at least a totally different form of treatment. Some doctors find it difficult to support the arbitrary decision-making process on who will receive interferon and who won't. They feel that the drug's worth can be shown by the accumulation of positive results in recipients, without necessitating the negative response of a control group.

"In this case it seems cruel and unnecessary," one researcher said. "What is the use for a cancer control group, other than statistics. If we give a cancer patient nothing, we know he'll die and we can predict when. We can do the same thing with known forms of treatment. If interferon's performance is significantly better, we'll be able to tell without using controls. I think we have a moral obligation to give the drug to everyone we possibly can."

More conservative scientists, though, are opposed to this view. They feel that formal and controlled studies are needed to wipe away any doubts about interferon. In Britain, the world's first major series of formal, controlled interferon trials are just now getting underway.

"There is some evidence of anti-tumor activity," says Derek Burke, "and the sensible, responsible thing to do right now is to get some of the stuff and see if it works. There's enough evidence to make it worthwhile spending a fair amount of money on this, if it's done properly."

Walter Bodmer explains that the design of the British series is a mixture. "I think the primary design is to see whether you get an effect of regression in the tumor. And, in the course of doing that, you want to look at all the effects that the drug has and what might be the most likely biological (cause of action). That can then allow you to better design further trials with the material to see how its effects might be mediated."

Cancer research, states Burke pointedly, is not like other research which might require only the necessary financial investment. "The process must be painstaking and constant. If you get a break, and interferon may be a break, you put money into it and spend five years finding out what you have. And, in the meantime, you keep basic research going, waiting for the next break to come. I think that's a very important scientific attitude. It's an attitude that's not widely understood because people think research advances are like putting somebody on the moon: you've only got to spend enough money. But that was the basis for President Kennedy's war on cancer, which really failed."

Norman Finter, who researches interferon for England's Burroughs-Wellcome pharmaceutical company, a major force in interferon work, explains the structure of the British program:

"When you develop a new drug, as a pharmaceutical company, you do it on a fairly rigid protocol. You learn how to make the drug, you check for purity, you carry out tests for safety which include laboratory tests and animal studies, monkey studies, and then you go into a first human trial. The first human trial, if you're going to do cancer patients, is what is called a Phase I study, which simply determines how much can be given for how long and what the side effects are. This is done in patients who have been asked to collaborate. They're told that it might do them some good, but it's not likely to; that it's not thought to do them any harm. We have done some of these studies with about thirteen patients, and we did find there was an upper safe limit to interferon use. If you give too much of it you get bone marrow depression and fever, but we also had objective evidence for tumor regression, so it was quite a nice result for a Phase I study.

"For this test, tumors weren't selected from any particular class. It was not looking for an anti-tumor effect. We just saw it fortuitously. That really reinforces the other anecdotal data that interferon is doing something. But until you do a controlled study all these things remain anecdotal. We didn't expect either of the responding patients to show these results. It was totally unexpected; these were fairly late cancer patients who had failed all other treatments and we were not expecting them to show spontaneous recovery. It was exciting in Phase I, but it's always conceivable it might have been just fortuitous.

"Our next step will be Phase II study in which you choose subjects either at random or on the basis of some previous experience. In this case we have some experience, categories of patients who are thought likely to show some response. For example, one is multiple myeloma, because published data shows that myeloma is highly fatal. We then look at the available existing treatments and make a decision as to whether it is ethical to give the new treatment against other patients who receive the best standard treatment or whether to give the new treatment plus the standard treatment. These are the same as in the testing of any other anti-cancer drug. Then it's laid out in such a way that the patients (a) know that they are taking part in a trial, but (b) they're not going to come to any clinical harm because it's not allowed that there would be a situation where they would be put in any jeopardy because they tried the new treatment."

That's all they're told. So their attitudes can't affect results. Only after these tests have been completed and evaluated will the British be completely satisfied that interferon performs. So stern is the British science community about this fact that one journal suggested: "Perhaps it would be quicker and kinder to cancer sufferers and their many relatives whose hopes have been stirred by interferon to call a halt to the small scale, anecdotal studies which, it could be claimed by the cancer sufferers, improve nothing more than the researcher's reputation."

These attitudes may seem harsh, but they mask a deep optimism about interferon's ultimate effectiveness. The British are simply afraid—especially after being tainted by the Glasgow hysteria—of promising too much, too soon; they want to be meticulous and sure. Still, Walter Bodmer speculates: "I would be surprised if in the long run interferon didn't turn out to be of some value in cancer therapy."

In America, Britain, and the rest of the cancer-phobic world, the public wants cancer eradicated. They want a cure. Scientists would love to find a cure, too. But they hold themselves on a tight rein and talk only in terms of improvement. They want to make cancer treatment better, safer, and less destructive to the patient. Many believe interferon will help them accomplish this goal, but there may be a price.

"You have to remember," says a major American interferon researcher, "that unless interferon turns out to be a total cure—all equally effective against all kinds of cancer, which doesn't seem likely given the variety and complexity of every facet of cancer development—then our determination of where it does work will also be a determination of where it doesn't work. Someone will be left out in the cold. And for that person the pain will be worse because so many others are helped."

The ultimate responsibility for accepting both interferon's blessings and its shortcomings, states the journal *Nature*, belongs with the individual. "To be sure, the enlightenment (about interferon) will not be comfortable news for all those who receive it. Some will learn that they may be denied the chance to benefit from some innovation. It is, however, entirely consistent with the temper of the times that people would have to learn to live with the painful knowledge that what happens to them, literally by fate, may be intrinsically determined by chance. Curiously enough, people were more ready to accept this hard truth in medieval times, no doubt because of their common conviction that heaven was, in any case, a better place. Now that circumstances have changed, more robust philosophies are needed."[3]

THE FUTURE OF TESTING

Despite such admonitions, desire for receiving interferon, experimental as it might be, remains tremendously high. And, happily, the research situation is entering a stage where many, many more patients will be able to become involved in the testing.

One researcher in the field states that in 1981 there will be "between 500 and 5000 times as much interferon" available as in previous years. The expansion in supply will bring a concomitant growth in testing. Odds are that the bulk of new experimentation will still center on the big cancer hospitals. They are simply better-equipped to put together patient populations and handle delicate drugs than small treatment centers or individual doctors.

The first impact of increased supply will be the expansion of research to more kinds of cancer. Patients whose cancers were excluded from the earlier tests will have a crack at interferon for the first time. The second growth area will be in the testing of new types of interferon. To date, all interferon used in human tests has come from processed human cells. By summer of 1981, however, significant amounts of interferon genetically engineered by bacteria whose cells have been altered by scientists will hit the research market.

In lab evaluations this non-human substance reacts just like human interferon. Soon after it becomes available, it will be tested on people to see if the lab results hold up. It will need to be compared with human interferon to see if the natural substance outperforms the genetically engineered versions. It will, in short, need all the evaluations human interferon has, plus a number of new ones.

All this work will require new experimental subjects. The number of patients involved in cancer tests with interferon could easily grow by a factor of ten within the next twelve to eighteen months.

Even at this level, however, interferon doesn't approach universal availability. The number of people who will become involved in testing will still be less than one percent of those who suffer from the disease. But there will be new openings for patients, and the best way to keep informed about any that might apply to a particular individual is by putting this person in touch with the nearest major cancer treatment center.

The most effective way to get in touch with the research institution is through the individual's private physician. No one is accepted into a drug experiment on their own word. Experimenters will always ask for the person's official medical record and talk with his doctor about the case. So the best place to begin investigating the possibility of joining a new interferon treatment program is in the personal doctor or cancer specialist's office.

It's possible that the details of some people's cases will instantly eliminate them from consideration for testing. The personal doctor should know about these conditions and should be able to explain why they make the patient a poor bet for testing. In other instances, the protocols of the new tests may stand against a given person's hopes of being admitted to the programs. These, too, can be discussed with and checked by a private doctor.

If it looks like there's a chance the person qualifies for an interferon test, the doctor should get in touch with the cancer center. He can talk the researchers' language and answer the detailed medical questions they'll ask before accepting anyone.

And then, a patient who does not get accepted must remember that there is little to cry about. Being turned down for interferon testing is not synonymous with being refused necessary aid. It's more like being turned away from a blackjack table in Las Vegas. If you had played, you had some chance to win, a bigger chance to lose; by not playing, at least you know you'll keep the money in your pocket.

As for today's gamblers with interferon, some win and some lose. But so strange is cancer testing that even the losers may actually have won something in the process.

Edward Tyler, for example, showed little response to interferon during his two month term on Gutterman's program. But, as he points out, "Who knows? The treatments didn't make my tumor any smaller during the test, but I'm still here. I still have a good appetite. Who knows what I would have been like without interferon. Maybe keeping me where I was really was a positive response."

Helen De Rise's case was more dramatic. "It had an immediate positive effect," she states. "It held my skin lesions in place but it did amazing things to the deeper tumors under the skin. It felt remarkable. I saw lumps I had had for months and months and months flatten out and disappear."

Peter DiFilippo still has his cancer, and still has his pluck. He recently went home to Washington, D.C., and got married. "It's hard to judge his case," says Dr. Susan Krown, "the treatment didn't shrink his tumor, but it did seem to flatten out the course of his disease, and he does seem to be holding up well since treatment. Cancer doesn't follow a highly predictable path. It's always full of dips and bumps. But I'd say overall the interferon probably did him some good."

Whatever their reactions, the recipients remain firmly convinced that interferon represents the path toward cancer treatment's future. "Even though it didn't shrink my tumor," says Tyler, "I remain convinced that interferon will cure cancer in certain circumstances and with certain cancers. I still think it has great promise and I'm very excited about it. I think it may cure one cancer or another within a year or two."

And Helen De Rise states that she would take interferon over any other form of treatment she could get today, whatever its drawbacks, and despite all that is not known about it. "I'd take it because, even though they don't know much, I feel that interferon has to be the way of the future. Compared to chemotherapy, which rolls right over you taking all the life right out of you, interferon is far preferable."

chapter 6

A TWO-EDGED SWORD

6

"I was very tired," says Edward Tyler, "just dog damn tired all the time. After I took my shot in the morning I just didn't have the energy to do anything. I couldn't walk with a brisk pace like I used to. So there's no question that interferon had side effects for me, but in comparison to some of the other stuff I've been through, it was nothing."

One of interferon's greatest attributes has been its relative lack of devastating side effects. Unfortunately, for many years the mildness of observed reactions against the protein became translated in many people mind's into a total absence of negative traits. By unequivocally stressing the positive, many doctors, quite unintentionally, left the public with an impression that interferon was the wonder drug that could cure without exacting any price.

It is one of nature's quirks, however, that no benefit derives without cost. There is no free lunch in medication, as in the environment. If a medication works on the body, it has to have side effects. By definition, an effective medication changes the functioning of some part of the body. Since bodily systems are intricately intertwined, any sort of change anywhere in the body will have rippling effects throughout the system. Some may be major, some almost unnoticable; but they will be present.

In the early days of interferon testing, the dosages used were so low they barely elicited a positive response, let alone a negative one. And the bedrock experiments were designed away from side effects and toward determining possible benefits of the drug. After all, it doesn't make much sense to use some of a rare precious substance to discover limitations before you've found out whether there's anything you want to use it for.

In those initial tests, virtually no side effects were noticed. Aspirin might produce the same amount of noticable activity. This helped create the image of interferon as being trouble free. More recently, however, dosages have begun to increase, and the number of patients being treated has risen. Also, some researchers are now turning exclusively to the question of side effects, since interferon clearly is headed for use in humans.

Unsurprisingly, indications of the drug's drawbacks have begun to emerge. The very potency of the protein requires that it create body-wide changes. The long- and short-term results of those changes have led Dr. Thomas Merigan to warn that "interferon can be a double-edged sword."

"It was a little naive," says Derek Burke, "that many of the people who were working on interferon came to believe that it was totally non-toxic, the universally beneficial substance. No substance, no matter how worthwhile, can be without its limitations and drawbacks."

One quirk in interferon studies was that scientists couldn't be sure that the interferon in their impure biological soups was actually causing any side effects they saw. It might have been the result of any of the hundreds of trace chemicals in the dross. Only now, with pure interferon becoming more available, can these doubts be laid to rest.

However, the weight of evidence so far indicates that it is, indeed, the interferon that creates side effects. A few of the offshoots grow milder as the purity of preparations grows stronger, but most of them seem to worsen when more interferon is present.

INTERFERON MALAISE

The effects felt most clearly by the interferon recipient form a lethargic condition that has been dubbed *interferon malaise.* After about a week of interferon treatments, many patients lose energy. They don't want to eat, they don't want to do anything. They might flop down for long, numbing naps, or get depressed easily.

The power of the malaise varies from patient to patient. Some interferon recipients bypass it entirely, for reasons scientists still don't understand. Many patients manage to continue working and getting through their normal activities, in spite of the periodic weakness. But others have to take to their beds while undergoing treatment.

Jim Beatty, one of the patients in Thomas Merigan's study of interferon and chronic hepatitis, suffered the malaise, but managed to get through a trip to England while self-administering doses of the protein. His vacation wasn't without its problems, however:

"I was very tired. I tended to keep going anyway, kind of a thing of will, and I did my mid-afternoon collapse every day. Nap is a nice way of putting it. I just stop and can't function for about two hours. Was I able to tolerate it? Well, I went to the opera every night, sometimes I went to sleep during act two, though."[1]

Interferon supporters point out that the malaise is a far less destructive condition than those wrought by chemotherapy and radiation. On the other hand, some patients who have received both treatments have said that they would just as soon get violently ill a few days each month than be totally listless every day.

In many interferon recipients, the malaise's effects aren't just physical. Their minds become involved as well. "It has been so strange," says Helen De Rise. "I have watched tumors go down and I can't get excited about it. In fact, I've felt incredibly depressed while on interferon. Others I know in the program feel the same way. I just feel incredibly sad and lonely, like I was treading water all by myself someplace. I feel like I'm waiting, waiting for something to happen, and I don't know what it is."

De Rise doesn't think her depression is mere disappointment at still having cancer. "This feels physical," she states. "It's hard to explain but I can't shake the feeling that it's somehow tied to the drug."

INTERFERON DAMAGE

More ominously still, studies are beginning to reveal subtler, but potentially more serious interferon effects that take place in the body organs and cells. The leader in uncovering interferon's hidden negatives has been Ion Gresser, the researcher who uncovered the protein's anti-cancer potential. He reviews the thinking that led him to study the drug's dark side: "We began thinking, as the known effects of interferon grew, that interferon is a very powerful biologic substance that slows down cell division and has different effects on the cells. Like all biologic substances that are very potent there may be instances where too much of it might not be good, we figured. This is so with all hormones. If you give too much estrogen or too much cortisone or any biologic material, you get bad effects. We wanted to know what the bad effects of interferon would be, because most people said that it's an anti-viral substance that has no bad effects. We showed that it did, indeed, have side effects.

"We decided to take newborn mice, because they're in a state of rapid growth, and see what happens. We treated them with interferon from the time they were born and showed that if you give them enough interferon for a week, you kill them with interferon. They die of liver necrosis. And then we found out that even if you stop the treatment before they die and they seem to recover, they develop kidney disease later in life.

"In addition, we found there is a virus in mice that causes the same type of disease as giving too much interferon and we were then able to show that in fact, the disease caused by this virus is not the result of the virus itself, it's because the virus makes a lot of interferon in the mice and the interferon kills them.

"So the interferon, instead of helping the mice in this particular example, does them in. The only point of this story is to say that interferon is usually beneficial; all our work shows that it is really an extremely useful and beneficial substance. But it has to be used with care because it is a very potent substance, and if you don't know what you're doing you can end up killing the mouse instead of saving it. That's the moral of the story," Gresser said.

In other words, Gresser showed that too much interferon can be deadly to mice. And a less than lethal dose of interferon can create health problems for the mice later in life. Curiously, he even discovered that, under the proper circumstances, interferon itself can bring on conditions that ape virus infections.

The key to this situation seems to be dosage. In a recent study subjecting mice to a high dose of interferon from their day of birth onward, the poor creatures died on their eighth day. A control group, given ten times less interferon, suffered no such fate. The reason why high doses of interferon may have destructive effects remains unclear, but worrisome.

Another question that is being raised about interferon use concerns its effect on antibody production. Norman Finter explains: "This situation is really quite paradoxical and hard to explain. Depending on the amount of interferon you give and the timing, you can either enhance or depress antibody formation. Generally speaking, it seems to depress antibody formation. But if you have an immunization schedule in progress, for example, and you then give it, you can sometimes enhance the function. The best course really does seem to be that you should give interferon before you give the antigen."

Uncertainty about antibody response means that interferon treatment could conceivably spur an attack of a disease or depress the functioning of antibodies already in the body, depending upon how and when it's given. This could limit the times and situations in which the protein could be used.

Interferon has shown disturbing power over certain liver enzymes as well, particularly in babies. Three of six human infants treated with interferon were found to have developed elevated levels of one important liver enzyme. The raised level didn't seem to cause any serious damage to the infants, and went away after treatment, but considering the severe liver damage shown by lab mice overdosed with interferon, the possibility exists that the protein may have a dangerous interaction with the liver. So far, the liver effect has been seen only in infants, not adults. This may mean either that the effect is greater in youngsters, or that it takes longer to show itself in bigger people.

The ties between interferon and individual cells hold the greatest perils for long-term treatment, just as they hold the greatest promise. Interferon takes over cells; it modulates their action, slows their division, and transforms their internal chemistry. In the natural situation, these changes are very temporary. But regular interferon treatments will keep some cells in the altered state more or less perpetually. What unhappy side effects might this cause?

Ion Gresser points up one: "Interferon can enhance or inhibit an immune response, and in some autoimmune diseases one finds interferons in the serum—but for the moment we don't know whether they actually are involved in the production of this disease." Autoimmune diseases are those in which the body's defenses turn against normal tissue, mistakenly identifying it as an invasive virus or bacteria. The protective immune cells attack and destroy their fellow body bits in an errant attempt to protect the host. Arthritis, lupus, and scleroderma are among the diseases now considered to be of autoimmune origin. There is some thought that interferon may sometimes provoke asthma attacks in certain people.

If long-term exposure to interferon can confuse the immune system into attacking normal cells, interferon recipients might be compromising their potentially pain-free senior years in exchange for a benefit today. Interferon treatment could even prove fatal in extreme cases.

Another worrisome trait of the potent protein is its apparent ability to depress the production of bone marrow. Bone marrow is responsible for creating blood cells and the platelets that help rid blood of infection. When interferon is present, the rate of cell division in the marrow drops. As a result, white blood cell counts drop. The same thing occurs during chemotherapy treatments.

This situation can leave an interferon recipient less able to fight off infections, since his platelet patrol is depleted, and often anemic, since the marrow isn't making as many red blood cells. Blood clotting may also be adversely affected, since the platelets play a role here, too.

In tests so far, at relatively low doses of interferon, all these changes have disappeared once the treatments have stopped. No one is certain how long they may last following a sustained treatment at a high dosage, however.

CREATING SAFEGUARDS

All of these foreboding potentials don't add up to a hopeless picture for interferon, however. Quite the contrary, like military leaders who have to think about the Bomb, biological researchers have to examine, soberly, the deadliest aspects of any substance they work with. Everything can be lethal under specific circumstances. When and where a medication falls on this shaded list is of paramount importance; it gives researchers an idea of a drug's relative safety and flexibility.

The more specifically negative aspects of the drug warn researchers about potential trouble situations, where the drug might cause more problems than it will solve. They also help the doctors formulate the best way to use the new drug, striking a balance between greatest possible effect and maximum safety.

Dr. Mathilde Krim, for example, notes that interferon's debilitation of the white blood cells doesn't mean that the drug can't be used, rather that "you might have to schedule the doses of interferon with rest periods between, to give the bone marrow a chance to recover. Bone marrow toxicity is a real problem; it's recognized and people are working on ways around it."

Kari Cantell manages to be both cautious and optimistic about the protein's drawbacks: "It is not impossible that the expanding clinical use of interferon may bring unpleasant surprises. Special caution is warranted whenever treatment with interferon is started in a new disease.

"As with any other medical treatment, when the risks of interferon treatment are considered, the beneficial effects must be weighed against the adverse effects. A determining factor in such an assessment is, of course, the nature of the disease to be treated. Both the common cold and rabies are viral infections. Both a wart and osteosarcoma are human tumors. But the acceptable risks in the treatment of these diseases differ greatly. Surprisingly, this obvious point has not been clearly understood when, for example, the question of a cell substrate for interferon production has been discussed. In the near future, interferon will not be used, like a vaccine, for the prophylactic treatment of large numbers of healthy people. It will be used for the treatment of already existing severe diseases."

And, the conclusion must be that the benefits of treatment will have to outweigh the possible side effects.

Derek Burke sees the picture of interferon's growing side effects as "an interesting theoretical question. It argues for caution in using large doses of interferon and for careful monitoring of patients. You can't use the completely theoretical argument about something being dangerous to keep you from trying a substance which might be effective against viruses and cancer. You just have to go ahead; you can't stop. But the possibility does argue for caution. It's a bit like gene cloning, where we've really realized the risks involved after taking great initial precautions, and people now have calmed down. The work went forward, but you had to take great precautions. With interferon, all these clinical trials are watched like a hawk's prey. But our fears should never keep them from being run.

"And then we get to the more philosophical question of whether our tampering can improve on the complex system nature gave us. It's certainly fallible because we all wear out and die, don't we? But I think it's wonderously made. We can accept that it's perfectly ethical to restore the hormone balance which has gone wrong, and which might create disorders of the thyroid or sex glands. But when it comes to interferon, we are talking about a substance that seems to be tied intimately into the entire system. By altering interferon's actions are we tearing the delicate web nature has built up?

"We don't know. We can only make our best effort to improve a diseased situation and watch things as carefully as possible to catch any untoward effects we might have brought into the system."

PART TWO

STORY OF A WONDER DRUG

chapter 7

UPWARD FROM MISINTERPRETATION

7

Attention to interferon seems unusually sudden. All at once, there is a wonder drug to fight cancer, when before there had been none and little hope of any. The irony is that interferon was discovered twenty-four years ago.

Unfortunately all the public usually sees of science is the splash and cacophony of the appearance of most advances. Most of us never see the steady, gradual drift upward toward light. That is why scientists are seldom as startled by the important developments in their fields as the public and the press. They have watched them coming for years. In science, as in show business, there really is no such thing as an overnight sensation.

In the summer of 1956, thirty-two year old Swiss researcher, Jean Lindenmann, came to work at England's National Institute for Medical Research in Mill Hill, near London. He had arrived for a one-year fellowship under the direction of Professor Christopher Andrewes, director of the Institute, in order to flee the repressive atmosphere of Zurich's Hygiene Institute, where a sixty-five year old curmudgeon ruled researchers with an iron fist and a firmly-fixed, backward gaze.

Lindenmann had become fascinated by the new field of virology—the study of those mysterious and destructive bits of genetic material that spawned diseases for which there was no cure. The miracle antibiotics that were the period's scientific pinnacle had no effect on the virus infections. Lindenmann wanted to help unravel the cloak of ignorance surrounding viral phenomena. Faced with the implacable enthusiasm of the young researcher, the set-in-his-ways administrator suggested a fellowship at some other institution where virology might be more fondly considered.

So Lindenmann cast about and eventually landed a year-long Swiss Fellowship to work in Mill Hill. His first task upon arrival was a futile attempt to grow polio virus in rabbit kidney cells, but he was so excited to be in England—where basic research wasn't looked upon as insanity—that the failure barely bothered him. It was thrilling for a young scientist to get his first taste of research in the beginning days of a totally new field of scientific inquiry. And on top of this, the institute was a world-renowned scientific center. Influenza virus had been discovered there in 1933. Lindenmann felt, for the first time in his career, that he had been called to the heartlands of scientific discovery. For the first time he was free of the mundane diagnostic chores he had been saddled with in Switzerland; he could research and learn all day long.

Despite his age, Lindenmann was still fairly naive in the scientific, if not the personal sense. The son of a railroad worker of Swiss extraction and his French-descended wife, Lindenmann was born in Zagreb, Yugoslavia, where his father had gone for engineering work. He led a nomadic early life—four years in Zagreb, then two years in Romania, then France, then back to Yugoslavia.

In Yugoslavia, Lindenmann developed lung tuberculosis and was sent back to stay in Switzerland. It was 1939, the eve of the Second World War. Lindenmann was fifteen. When the war broke out, his parents were trapped in occupied Yugoslavia while he went through high school and college in Zurich.

Perhaps because of his personal experience with the ravages of infection, Lindenmann centered his studies on microbiology, particularly the understanding of the roots of disease. Eventually, this interest broadened to include the little understood role of viruses.

The man crafted by Lindenmann's early life was scientifically sharp, but diffident and shy. He had somehow retained an almost boyish glee in science, but was ill-suited to the politics and power plays of a major scientific institute. He still felt that research involved noble scientists in the search for verities that would help their fellow humans. When creative scientists were free to follow their informed speculations, he believed that marvelous insights and exciting discoveries could follow.

Unfortunately, this was not the case at the Institute in Zurich. Disillusioned but buoyant, Lindenmann went to England with high hopes. The research situation was close to his ideal of selflessness and free-minded investigation, but he felt hampered by his weak command of English and somewhat overpowered by the ambition and scientific clout of those around him.

One friendly person went out of his way to make the unassuming Swiss researcher feel comfortable at Mill Hill. He was a strongly featured, darkly handsome Englishman who worked in a different section of the giant lab. He would join the younger researcher for tea and pleasant conversation, drawing him out, establishing a warm, cordial spot that Lindenmann came to look forward to.

His name was Alick Isaacs and he was one of the most renowned biologists in the United Kingdom. Though Isaacs, thirty-five, was not much older in years than Lindenmann, he had already carved an important place for himself in the history of English virology. Throughout the 1940s, Isaacs worked in England and later in Australia to discover basic facts about the influenza virus, whose apparently infinite variety of forms eluded any decent sort of prevention. The study of this epidemic-spreading virus comprised the bulk of Isaac's career, and brought him most of his scientific fame. Interferon grew from a side avenue in Isaacs's interest, almost a hobby—his fascination with the question of viral interference.

The question that haunted Isaacs while he worked at influenza studies was why a person who is stricken by one virus is virtually never stricken by a second simultaneously. What is the mechanism by which one virus interferes with another?

It wasn't a new question. Back in the nineteenth century, Erasmus Darwin, grandfather of the naturalist Charles Darwin who would later develop the theory of natural selection, realized that he had never seen one of his patients recovering from measles who had contracted the dreaded smallpox. At the time, of course, he had no idea that both diseases were caused by viruses and interference was involved. He merely wondered why.

That query echoed through work over the next half century. In 1937, G. W. M. Findlay and F. O. MacCallum of Great Britain found that monkeys infected with Rift Valley fever virus were somehow protected from the fatal effects of yellow fever virus. They knew that the protection could not have been caused by antibodies because antibodies developed by the body to fight Rift Valley fever virus have no effect on yellow fever virus. Findlay and MacCallum coined the term "virus interference" for their discovery. They believed that when one virus invaded a group of cells, a second virus was excluded. But they didn't know how. Later, laboratory studies using fertilized hens' eggs and tissue cultures demonstrated that virus interference was a common occurrence. In 1943, Werner and Gertrude Henle, working at the Children's Hospital of Philadelphia, found that viruses killed by gentle heat or ultraviolet light could still interfere with the growth of other viruses.

But for two decades after Findlay and MacCallum described virus interference, the specifics of its functioning defied explanation. Why and how did infection of a cell by one virus prevent infection by a second?

In 1948, Isaacs received a fellowship to spend a year working at the Walter and Elize Hall Institute in Melbourne. At the end of that term, he got a second grant to stay another year. He wished to stay because the progress he and his partner, Margaret Edney, had made at unravelling viral interference was exhilarating.

Using chicken eggs, they performed a wide range of experiments that drew the first parameters for the performance of interference. They showed that one virus could block the functioning of several others, that a minimum dose was required for interference to begin, and that whatever was going on took place inside the infected cells.

Unfortunately, Isaacs and Edney still could not pin down the nature of the interference function. Their first thought was that the two viruses must somehow be battling against one another for vital cell components. But this conclusion was wrong.

In 1951, Isaacs returned home to take a prestigious post with the National Institute for Medical Research at the World Influenza Center. Soon after Isaacs began work at the influenza center, a widespread flu epidemic began. He provided evidence that the viruses reaching Britain in 1951 were of two origins. Some, the Scandinavian strains, apparently arose as activations of infection which had been dormant since the previous winter and had then reached Britain across the North Sea, while others, the so-called Liverpool strains, probably came from the Southern hemisphere. Isaacs found that most viruses south and west of a line from Ireland to Italy were like 'Liverpool', those to the north and east were 'Scandinavian'. Drawing on this case study, Isaacs developed a picture of how flu spreads. 'Flu outbreaks', he determined rarely spread indefinitely but ultimately peter out: that outbreaks tend to arise on the fringes of past epidemics, where 'emerging' viruses may find less hindrance from widespread immunity.

Isaacs backed this work with a wide assortment of studies on every facet of influenza, flu outbreaks, and the history and function of this sweeping disease. Looking back, influenza research might not seem too riveting. But in the 1950s, remember, our understanding of viruses was scant and the impact of flu was far greater than it is today. Scientists had no means at the time to identify flu strains quickly and prepare huge batches of vaccine. They could only watch the approaching epidemic and try to warn the public it was coming. Much of our ability today to cope with flu stems directly from the work of Isaacs and the other virologists of his time.

While the main thrust of his work expanded our understanding of flu, Isaacs never lost his incessant curiosity about viral interference. He fell into the habit of using visiting fellows at the Institute to run after-hours studies of various interference problems. Throughout the 1950s, these teams produced results that indicated strange and potentially important properties of interference between viruses. But they brought Isaacs no closer to finding the nexus of the process. He still didn't know what interference was.

One day during tea, Lindenmann and Isaacs talked about viral interference. It turned out that the year before Lindenmann had tried an interference experiment of his own. It had been only partially successful, but it piqued Isaacs's interest.

"How did you deactivate your viruses?" he asked Lindenmann, concerning an intricacy of test method.

"By the method of two Australians, Isaacs and Edney," Lindenmann replied placidly, using a homegrown pronunciation of the names which kept him from realizing he was sitting across the table from the man who had invented the method. Only after Isaacs had shot a series of piercing, wry questions at him did he realize what was up. Without knowing it he had paid Isaacs a compliment. Perhaps this helped generate the professional interest that drew the pair into mutual experiments. In any case, during the fall of 1956, Isaacs had Lindenmann freed from his other chores and set him up to perform experiments in viral interference.

As happens so often in science, what Lindenmann and Isaacs were looking for and what they found were far different. They wanted to examine interference, not so much for itself as to discover more about the basic functioning of viral infections. Figuring out the process that blocked them might help explain how they progressed. The pair began with the hypothesis that viruses were something like bacteriophages—protein sacks with their nucleic acids inside. The sacks attached to cells and injected their genetic information into the cell material, leaving an empty envelope attached to the cell wall.

They set up their first experiment to show that viruses attached to red blood cells left their empty husks behind and that this might be the reason for interference. It flopped. The first step of the test produced information so uncertain and confusing it made any further attempts useless.

In the meantime, the team arranged another experiment with much the same preliminary question in mind: Could the virus-coated red blood cells' power to induce interference be exhausted by prolonged contact with egg membranes, and could the virus be revealed in the fluid as an interfering entity? They let virus-coated red cells induce interference in a set of membranes. Then they removed the membranes, washed off the red cells, and added them to a second set of membranes. At the same time, they placed fresh membranes into the fluid from the first experiment. The result of this experiment revealed a totally different interference situation: The red cells, as expected, again induced interference; but the fluid alone also induced interference. Why? Attempts to neutralize the interfering activity with anti-viral antiserum, or to bring it down by high-speed centrifugation failed.

At that moment, the concept of interferon was born. Around November, 1956, Alick Isaacs, in his small tidy handwriting, wrote in his notebook: "In search of interferon." This word, which Lindenmann had initially coined as a joke—witticisms, as has been said, were infectious around Isaacs—soon became an accepted term.

What Lindenmann and Isaacs had begun to suspect was that interference was not a reaction of virus against virus, but the result of the emergence of a cell-produced substance. It was a startling thought in those days; the currently accepted notions of cell complexity and systems-thinking came to the fore in biology more recently. They knew they had found something in the biological soup of the cell fluid, but they weren't sure what it was. Something in those very impure soups inhibited the growth of a second virus, but the experimenters had no idea whether it was one substance or several substances. But they knew it must be something material, because heating as well as other manipulations could destroy it. At one point quite near the beginning of their work, they suddenly thought maybe it was not the presence of something but the lack of something. Maybe a nutrient was being used up in the culture system, thus preventing the second virus from growing. If that had been true, interferon would not have been any more than the lack of something. They nearly panicked at the thought of discovering something that wasn't there, but they pressed on to determine what it was they had stumbled upon.

To find out whether they were right in assuming interferon was a substance, the pair devised an experiment that has become a modern classic. It exemplifies the qualities of simplicity, elegance, and irrefutability that any good test should have. And it shows how scientists can use the same techniques, with a slightly different twist, to transform failed experiments into masterpieces.

Like their other tests, Lindenmann and Isaacs began this one by deactivating a virus through heating it, the process that Isaacs had developed in Australia. But this time, they dispensed with any human blood cells or other additional experimental ingredients. The entire experiment was with the chick membranes they had used earlier.

Strips of the living membrane were placed in neutral culture fluid and exposed to the deactivated virus. The process has been described as creating "a battleground in a test tube." Isaacs and Lindenmann believed that the cell's battle against the virus would release whatever substance it was that caused interference.

After sufficient time passed for the battle to be waged, the team took fresh shell membranes and exposed them—not to the virus—but to the virus-free fluid of the infected cells in their first batch. When this second set of membranes was exposed to a new virus, it resisted. Interference had occurred. Something created by the beseiged cells in the first batch—not the virus itself—had protected the cells of the second batch from viral infection. Isaacs and Lindenmann had proven the existence of interferon.

The pair's 1957 paper on their discovery created a scientific storm. When told about their work, Lindenmann's "old boss" back in Zurich wouldn't believe the findings. Others around the world felt the same way. American scientists dubbed the discovery "misinterpreton," convinced that Isaacs and Lindenmann had read into their results the findings they so deeply desired.

Others, however, hailed the new substance as the viral penicillin—the breakthrough that would rid the world of yellow fever and flu. The British science council felt enthusiastic enough about interferon to ask permission from the discoverers to request a patent in their names for the benefit of future research.

"The term 'breakthrough'," wrote Dr. C. H. Andrewes some years later, "is one of the most abused and overworked especially in popular accounts of science, but it can justly be used concerning the discovery of interferon."

The skeptics of those early days shouldn't be scorned, however, states Dr. Samuel Baron, an interferon researcher from nearly the beginning. "It's fair and honest to say that most scientists must be skeptical in order to sort out truly valid findings from those not so valid. Just before interferon was announced, several natural substances had been announced as effective against viruses that were not as effective as they had been thought to be. Interferon met with the same skepticism, even more in fact. Scientists wanted to see more data before being convinced."

Baron, in fact, had entered interferon research as a doubter. When he came to Mill Hill, he was dismayed to be told he was going to work on the new discovery. "I was a little put back by that suggestion, but I thought about it and finally said, 'yes, I'm willing to give it a try.' The next morning, I went into Alick Isaacs's lab and found that Alick was away on vacation in Denmark. His research assistant and I sat down and I said, 'prepare me some of this and let's see how it works.' By the end of the week I was completely convinced. I found interferon completely protects cells against otherwise lethal viruses."

SETBACKS

In the best of all possible worlds, interferon would have marched a swift and stately course to scientific prominence, while Lindenmann and Isaacs would have risen to riches and acclaim. But it didn't work out that way. Following the initial burst of excitement, interest in interferon began to fade away.

At the end of his fellowship, Jean Lindenmann left Mill Hill and returned to Switzerland. He felt the development of interferon was now a matter for technicians and would not take much time. They could figure out how to make it and test it in the laboratory. As a biologist rather than a lab specialist, he felt his best role would be a few years later when purified preparations of interferon would become available. He had no idea that it would be more than twenty years before that stage would be reached.

Isaacs took on new assistants, Samuel Baron and Britisher Derek Burke, and plowed ahead into interferon study. He and his team began to sketch in the characteristics of the newly discovered substance. They ran through the accepted scientific tests for establishing what a substance is made of and how it operates. Derek Burke recalls the time:

"It went very well for the first few months. Everything we did was new, everything we did was publishable. Then we started running into problems and the pace of work began to slow down. We were making chick interferon that wouldn't work in mouse cells or human cells. We needed to make interferon active in humans and that took rather a long time."

"What went wrong," Burke feels, "was that it was very hard to capitalize on the first human experiment, which showed that interferon blocked a virus when injected into a human arm. That was an important experiment and we thought it would be fairly easy to move into other human situations. Actually, it took ten years. And there were a lot of failed experiments during those ten years.

"In retrospect I'd have to say it was because we didn't have enough knowledge. We had no idea how highly potent interferon was. We had no tools to disentangle the system. We really knew very little about it. Right through the 1960s it was a very messy field.

"And, sad to say, Alick oversold how easy it would be. He kept saying, Well, we'll do this and then it will work, and it didn't work. There were several negative studies in the 1960s which weren't published, but which influenced the disposition of money and basically the pharmaceutical firms decided that interferon wasn't going to work."

Lindenmann remembers being at a meeting once in 1962, five years after interferon was discovered. There was some discussion where interferon was mentioned, and someone said "well, interferon has now been talked about for the last five years, and if it were really something, we would know by now." There was a tendency at this time to negate interferon's existence; it was a difficult subject because you could not come up with the pure substance and say, "this is it, it works."

Interest in interferon plummeted when it was found that the

protein was species specific. It would require human interferon to achieve results in people, and scientists at the time knew of no sound procedure for getting interferon from human cells.

The protein was stymied by lack of knowledge. It was, in fact, discovered before its time. From 1957 through the early 1960s, the science of virology was in a state of infancy. The most basic questions about what viruses were and how they worked were just being answered. Vast gaps in knowledge lay all over the field. It is scant wonder that finding a niche for interferon proved daunting, since there was really no framework in which to fit the drug.

Faced with so many unknown facts and unanswered questions, many virologists grew sharply impatient with interferon. If it wasn't going to be the miracle vaccine that would put the science on the map, then they had no time for it. If it showed problems and shortcomings, they had more important topics to address before they fooled around with a confusing, troublesome treatment.

Big-time science left interferon behind. It seemed just another botched virus cure, another experiment whose results promised too much. When Alick Isaacs died in 1967, interferon had only just begun to come out of this severe trough. Although his belief in the substance's value never diminished, he, like many discoverers before him, didn't live to see his belief fulfilled.

Lindenmann, meanwhile, had moved from job to job, a nomad once again. He spent a couple of years in Bern, took a professorship in Florida State University at Gainesville, and finally returned to the Institute in Zurich. His old boss had retired.

Let's consider the elusive process by which scientific discoveries are made and promoted. At the time he joined Isaacs, Lindenmann didn't feel anything special was going on; this was how normal science should work, he believed. Looking back, though, he realized that it was a time and place where a very rare event occurred; the ability for strong minds to take a completely fresh look at an old problem was rare indeed. Here was a researcher willing to work himself to a frazzle. He was both enthusiastic and naive enough to try anything, and he had no preconceptions to limit his work. At one moment and place, this unique mind converged with that of an administrator and gifted scientific thinker, who had the clout to accomplish what he wanted, and the insight to define problems in solvable forms.

Asking which of the two was more important to the discovery

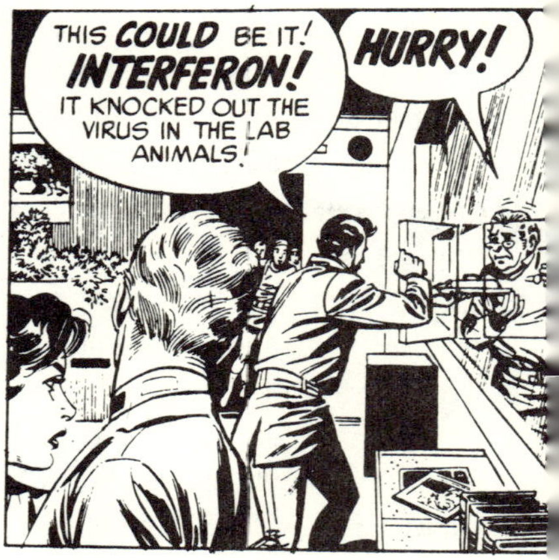
THIS COULD BE IT!
INTERFERON!
IT KNOCKED OUT THE
VIRUS IN THE LAB
ANIMALS!
HURRY!

The promise of interferon was seen as early as 1960 in this *Flash Gordon* comic strip. Here, space medics inject interferon to fight an extraterrestrial virus.

is unimportant. Like the lyricist and the composer, they were equally and uniquely indispensable to the process. They were the right personalities at the right place and at the right time asking the right question; and they were free enough to accept the answer they received, unexpected as it may have been.

From the viewpoint of the early 1960s, however, the moment of interferon's unveiling might not have seemed so propitious; the flame of interest had almost died. Only a small band of devotees kept thinking about, and working with, interferon. The fire was banked, not cold.

In all courses of discovery, there seem to be valleys, long periods when little overt happens. At the time, the search always appears to be dead, barren, and worthless. But in retrospect, these interludes turn out to be invaluable periods of consolidation. Nowhere can this be seen better than with interferon.

The Mill Hill experiments begat the interferon work of Samuel Baron and Derek Burke. Virtually simultaneous work in America created flurries of interferon interest that inspired Kurt Paucker and Ion Gresser. In 1962, Paucker saw something that looked suspiciously like an anti-tumor effect created by interferon. At about the same time, Gresser, who had moved to Paris, determined that human leukocytes—white blood cells—might provide a superior source for human interferon.

A young Finn, Kari Cantell, who had worked with Paucker in

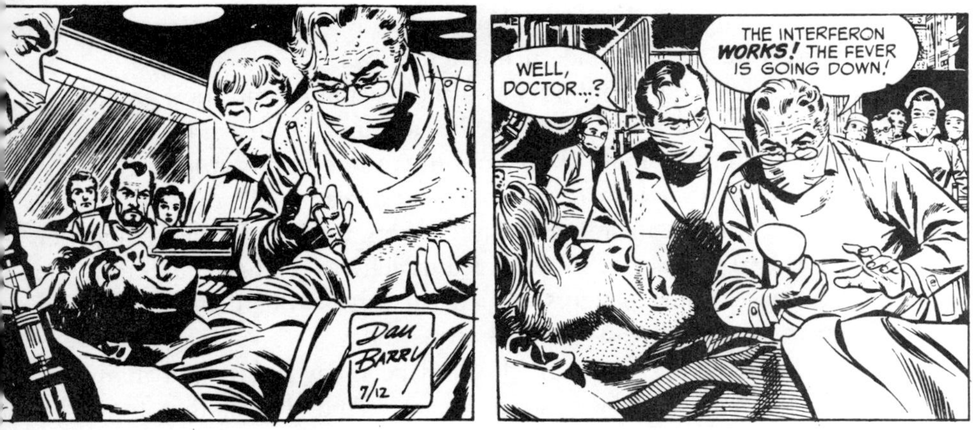
WELL, DOCTOR...?
THE INTERFERON WORKS! THE FEVER IS GOING DOWN!

Philadelphia, heard about Gresser's idea. He was favorably disposed toward interferon because of what he'd seen of it in the United States, and he knew something about leukocytes because he'd gone home to Helsinki to run his country's Public Health Blood Bank. Cantell began mulling over the possibilities of using his lab's leukocytes to make interferon.

Meanwhile, the few serious researchers, unable to get any human interferon and in need of funding money, spent their time on small animal studies. In 1965, Gresser revealed a clear-cut anti-tumor effect by interferon in mice. Barry Jones, at the Morefield Eye Hospital in England, tried topical applications of interferon on herpes infections that burned ulcers beside the eyes of rabbits.

No cure for the recurring disease was known at the time, but interferon made the ulcers disappear first in the rabbits, then in people.

ATTEMPTS AT PRODUCTION

As reports began to filter out of the interferon community about such results, interest slowly began to return to the maligned protein. But a serious roadblock still barred the path to interferon's scientific rehabilitation. Researchers needed to be able to get their hands on enough interferon for sufficient tests.

Cantell thought and tinkered, quietly creating the process that would usher in the modern interferon age.

Cantell's contribution was almost certainly the most important since interferon was discovered, because for the first time it ensured a steady, though small, supply of human interferon for testing. Without his persistence in trying to devise a reasonable method of production, interest in interferon might very well have faded altogether by the 1970s. Instead, his work led directly to the first interferon tests in human cancer patients, which, in turn, brought on the fevered interest in the protein that still grows today.

"Interferon," says Cantell, "has been my hobby and main scientific interest for over twenty years." And during that time, he searched with a diligence few scientists could match for the proper combination of ingredients to produce usable levels of interferon from human cells. He worked almost alone with no fanfare or outside support. Spurred by the fanaticism of the radical tinkerer, he simply refused to stop trying different possibilities until one worked.

The site where all this work took place is highly unspectacular—a small, drab suite of labs in Helsinki's Central Public Health Laboratory. It was to these labs that Cantell returned from America in the early sixties to take on the job of separating and purifying donor blood for Finnish hospitals. The process of preparing the blood for use in patients required that it be separated into component parts. Some 500 to 800 pints of whole blood flowed each day into Cantell's lab where it was spun in a centrifuge to separate the various types of cells.

Of primary importance to doctors were the heavy red blood cells which sank to the bottom of the centrifuge chamber. The other element doctors required was the thin liquid blood plasma which rose to the top of the separated blood. In between these two portions lay a thin layer of solid white cells—the leukocytes. In Cantell's and every other blood lab in the world, they were removed from the centrifuge and thrown away.

When Cantell heard of the possibility that leukocytes could produce large amounts of interferon, he realized that the situation afforded new possibilities. His existing lab setup already separated out the leukocytes, so he had an unending supply of them to test and toy with to see if interferon really could be gleaned from them.

Instead of tossing out the leukocytes, Cantell began to save them.

He literally rescued the interferon movement from the sewer. He created new kinds of lab glassware to do a better job of separating out the white blood cells. Then he devised a program for stimulating the cells to produce interferon.

Cantell began injecting his leukocytes into eggs. Then he would add a virus to the egg and incubate the mixture for twenty-four hours at just under 100 degrees. After each application, Cantell would use the centrifuge to separate the white cells from the fluid into which they had released their interferon. And he would test the resulting biological soup to see how much interferon was present.

In the beginning, Cantell achieved higher levels of interferon than anyone had in other kinds of cells, but still not enough to warrant a full-scale production facility. The viruses he was using didn't seem to provide the maximum level of interferon stimulation. He had no way to test interferon production except to try viruses by trial-and-error. And it seemed a depressing prospect. But instead of giving up, Cantell began testing a veritable chemical dictionary of viruses. He tried dozens of viruses that wouldn't be fatal to humans; the chance of contamination in the interferon kept him away from those. Every one he tried, though, was disappointing.

So little was known about interferon that it was impossible for Cantell to judge which viruses might generate the best effect. He was working in the dark on a purely trial-and-error quest. Finally, after several years, Cantell tried a fairly innocuous virus called Sendai. For the first time, his eggs spouted interferon, more than ten times as much as from any other virus. Cantell decided that he had found the right combination for producing interferon: Sendai virus and leukocytes.

The next step was the creation of an on-going production system. However, because of the requirements of working with leukocytes and eggs, Cantell had to keep his interferon factory small and personal. Machines couldn't handle the leukocytes or turn the eggs or carry them around the lab. It took people. So, even after he went into full-time interferon production, the operation was tiny and produced small amounts of the protein—barely enough for a couple hundred people to be treated a few weeks—at enormously high prices.

To understand the problems, consider the fact that a literal river of blood is required to produce one milligram of interferon. Forty thousand donors must give blood to produce enough interferon for just 150 patients. All of this blood has to be taken and separated, the leukocytes must be removed and purified. They are suspended in a culture medium and exposed to the Sendai virus, then incubated for 24 hours. The resulting mixture is centrifuged to separate the cells and virus from the interferon they have made. Each dose of interferon requires a flood of fresh blood; the leukocytes cannot be grown in lab cultures and can only be used once. The system is slow, wasteful, and round-about and it was the only system of any importance for years.

Cantell's process produced a trickle of interferon that cost—breathtakingly—between $70 and $100 per trillionth-of-a-gram. But at least he was producing a steady, reasonably reliable supply. For the first time, scientists had human interferon with which to work. Still, what Cantell was producing wasn't pure interferon. One researcher has described it as "leukocyte soup contaminated with minute amounts of interferon." Cantell's soup was only .1 per cent pure—999 parts of each unit were relatively harmless organic junk, leaving only one part interferon.

But this was better than nothing.

RESULTS

While Cantell was spending a decade poking around for the proper interferon combination, he was joined by a young Swedish physician, Hans Strander. The course of interferon's development in the phase following Cantell's initiation of production in 1970 shows again how a winding thread of curiosity, mutual interest, and happenstance draws scientific findings and ideas slowly but steadily forward. Strander begins the second chain.

After spending a few years working with Cantell, Strander went back home to Stockholm where he joined the Karolinska Hospital. He handled cancer patients, but one form of cancer affected him most profoundly: osteogenic sarcoma, a bone cancer which struck young people in their teens. Its course was swift, disfiguring, and almost always fatal. Because he knew about Cantell's work in Helsinki, Strander decided not to give up on these patients without at least trying some of the Finn's interferon. He figured it couldn't hurt, since their chances of surviving the tumor flare-up that usually followed amputation surgery were extremely thin. He gave several dozen of them interferon and about half fared well over two years, compared to an 85 percent fatality rate without the drug.

The enticing but quizzical results Strander reported in his informal tests with these unfortunate children filtered through the ranks of virologists, immunologists, and cancer physicians. The findings, insubstantial as they were, began to stimulate interest and action.

In New York, a cancer physician at Sloan-Kettering became convinced by the early 1970s that interferon held enough promise to be worth full-time investigation. She began to lobby hard for some sort of formal interferon program at the Sloan, but the road was not easy. Dr. Mathilde Krim recalls how she put her shoulder to the bureaucratic door and pushed for interferon:

"I've been interested in putting together a lab like the Interferon Evaluation Program since the early seventies. But, for many reasons there were delays and delays. Besides, there was no money then for interferon work. Finally, in 1974, a unit called "Interferon Evaluation Section" was created, and I was made the head of it, but I was alone. There was nobody else. For myself, I needed to know what had been learned firsthand. I made a kind of review of the evidence, particularly the chemical work, which had started in Sweden." Krim went to Sweden, to Finland, to France, to Switzerland, to learn as much about interferon research as could be learned. She decided that although evidence of human cancer successes in these programs was still small, interferon nevertheless became very enticing.

"Now in those days, one could hardly speak of an anti-tumor effect. We had no idea, for example, that we would see tumor regressions. We did not hope for that because in animals, in fact, regressions had not been seen. It was only an inhibition of growth, or lack of appearance of tumor. But the interferon was sufficiently interesting, in my opinion, just as an anti-viral, that I went to the National Cancer Institute and said, 'I think there is enough evidence to warrant your support in this field in addition to what you've been doing until now.' They wanted to protect their turf. They didn't want anyone else taking interferon out of their control."

In any case, the institute gave Krim a grant to organize an international workshop. "They said, fine, you may have a point, but we would like to hear it from more people, so let's bring all the experts together and do a review and evaluate where we're going in this field; where it really has promise." The first international workshop at Sloan-Kettering "was a hell of a good little meeting," according to Krim. "It was very exciting because it was the first time that everybody in the field was brought together. And, that outsiders were brought in too, who were in fields that would have an impact."

"One of them was our director, Dr. Goodrich, and I must say, to his credit, that he really was very open-minded. A few young people at the meeting who had worked in interferon before asked Dr. Goodrich to give them a lab here for interferon. He accepted. And, then, I was asked to organize the thing. That's how this lab started."

SCIENCE'S SEARCH FOR MONEY

One of those attending Krim's 1975 meeting was Dr. Jordan Gutterman, an immunologist from the M.D. Anderson Hospital in Houston, Texas. Here, for the first time, he heard about interferon as a potential tool against human cancer:

"Hans Strander's studies were first reported in 1975 at an international conference on interferon in New York at the Rockefeller Institute. That is where I first heard the results and I was very intrigued not only by the results Dr. Strander was achieving but about the whole possibility of using the various interferons in cancer patients. Here was a non-toxic substance, a natural substance, that not only stopped the growth of viruses but stopped the growth of cancer cells, and it seemed that this material was worthy of further work. The problem was simply one of money."

The enormous expense of interferon might have daunted other researchers, but not Gutterman. He scoured the country for an angel. "The cost of production was $150 per dose. The dose Dr. Strander was using was three million units a day—the same number of units we now use of this material. At $150 per dose—he was giving it on a daily basis—it would cost literally several thousand dollars to treat even one patient. The National Institutes of Health and the National Cancer Institute had looked at the situation and said there was very little clinical information and that it was too risky really to invest a large amount of money in further clinical work . . . Late in 1977, Mrs. Mary Lasker, who had been a major figure in the whole area of cancer research, gave a contribution to the M.D. Anderson Hospital and Tumor Institute to allow us to do initial testing in patients with advanced cancer."[1]

Gutterman's findings with Mrs. Lasker's money deepened his interest in interferon and gave him the courage to go to the American Cancer Society with a 135-page grant request for $2 million to buy more of the protein; this was the biggest single research request in the Society's history. When the Cancer Society decided to offer this grant, interferon exploded. After some twenty years in scientific diaspora, the drug had come back to the spotlight. And, ironically, on its second trip to the top, interferon appeared to show far greater powers than ever claimed for it by its discoverers. If they had ever raised the notion that interferon would become the great white hope of cancer research, they would have been ridiculed. In the case of interferon, patience among researchers was surely its own reward.

The leap of insight that occurred in the work of Lindenmann and Isaacs—in which interferon was discovered—came before science was ready to understand it. The case is similar to that of an architect who designs a building that builders aren't yet able to construct. It is as confusing as it might be admirable.

In 1957, science didn't know much about the genetic workings of cells. Virologists could barely explain the viruses themselves, let alone a trace substance that seemed to stop them in their tracks. Interferon eventually refound its niche in research, not just because of the researchers who stuck with it through the two lost decades, but because understanding in other fields managed to catch up. As Derek Burke states:

"Things picked up with interferon because advances in other fields helped us to work on interferon, advances in cell biology and genetics. All of a sudden we had much better purification methods. All of a sudden we could investigate how it kept viruses from multiplying. All of a sudden we had different sorts of cells to study interferon production in. All these things made it very much easier to really find out how it was made, what it was and how it worked."

Not only did ancillary sciences grow up around interferon, but the field of virology itself grew larger, more confident, and better able to attack thorny, uncertain problems like interferon. In the early days of interferon, virology had far more important matters on its mind. It had to establish the roots of the subject, and the basic definitions and concepts. What necessarily followed were the exciting early days of discovery and conjecture. When relationships between tumors and viruses appeared, they held the attention of many young virologists for several years. Vaccines needed to be formulated for polio, measles, flu, and other nasty viral diseases.

In a new field of study like virology, there is so much exciting work to be done and so few pioneers to handle the work that anything not of obvious, immediate benefit gets neglected for a time. But as the field grows, and as the number of scientists as a whole increases, old questions are answered, and more and more manpower becomes free to look around for new ones or dust off deserving old ones. The problem of polio—vaccine, diagnostics, population surveys—occupied several hundred virologists for years. When the basics of polio became known, and the groundwork was laid, many of these researchers were suddenly free to look around for ideas.

And for some, these ideas came in the field of viral causes of cancer and eventually interferon. And their work produced results that stimulated more and more work until suddenly the field was rejuvenated.

To the public, it appears that research work goes from a dead stop to a wild careen of activity; but to scientists it appears otherwise. They know that work has never really ceased. With interferon, in fact, publications gradually increased throughout the doldrum period. Movement was small but steady—a quiet development below the surface of public awareness. When the power of fresh work energized the field, it suddenly rose into public view like a surfacing submarine. Still, Derek Burke chides, "all the while people have been working, developing techniques that allowed us to ask questions about the interferon system which were quite impossible earlier."

If you want to climb a wall—one which is both dangerous and tall, and seemingly insurmountable—you first have to determine where to scale it. You might take considerable time pondering the move, testing various alternatives in your mind, and checking conditions at the site. Only after you have defined your needs could you do it.

Research is much the same. Most of the time and effort goes into determining what needs to be done, what problem must be overcome, where scientists must scale the fence of ignorance. Every few years, study on a topic reaches a point where a particular scientist or team are able to ask the right question and produce an experiment that takes understanding over the wall, and into new realms of speculation.

These leaps are the breakthroughs that most people see as the real role of research. In truth, they are the result of—as opposed to the reason for—genuine research. As the process goes, there is testing—definition—leap, then testing—definition—leap, then over and over again, each time moving slightly ahead, each time clearing up a question or raising a potentiality.

And that is how interferon has developed in its twenty-four-year history. For a long time, the searching was confused, the testing uncertain, and the leaps tiny. Now the search has grown more intense and the leaps are getting larger. But the basic process has never varied. Generally, it has worked this way in science for generations and probably will continue in like manner for even longer.

The most recent leap in the interferon story involves purity, the problem Kari Cantell couldn't solve. How could interferon be separated from its biological soup so that the effects of 100-proof substance could be determined? Everything scientists tried to cull from the interferon failed. But the work served to define the problem and eliminate directions that wouldn't work.

Finally, in the past year, Derek Burke came up with the answer, a monoclonal antibody. An antibody is a chemical that latches onto another chemical, rendering it impotent. Our bodies produce antibodies when they detect infections. The antibodies link with the invading agents, making it impossible for them to latch onto body parts. A monoclonal antibody is one that links exclusively with one other molecule.

Of Burke's discovery of a monoclonal antibody for interferon, Mathilde Krim says: "It is a momentous event, because a monoclonal antibody is a very highly specific antibody for a single species, unlike natural antibodies which are mixtures of reacting agents. And, secondly, this particular antibody can be produced in unlimited amounts because it comes from a cell growing in suspension. It can be made very cheaply, very easily. Every twenty-four hours the cells divide, and put out antibodies, so you can collect huge amounts and purify it efficiently."

With the antibody in hand, interferon producers can do a far better job of separating the protein from the soup. The antibody will link up with interferon and nothing else. Once the two have joined, removing the antibody means removing all the interferon as well. The resultant fluid is interferon and antibody, and nothing else. When the antibody is stripped off, all that's left is interferon.

The antibody also makes it possible to prove beyond any shadow of a doubt that the effects of the biological soup are caused by interferon and not some other unknown ingredient. If the soup creates an effect which stops when the antibody is added, then interferon must have produced it; it is the only substance the antibody will stop.

Burke's finding has greatly enhanced the possibilities for using genetically engineered interferon. And the scientific chain continues. It was the impending appearance of genetic engineering that lay in the background as interferon approached the crucial cusp of human testing. The likelihood of breakthroughs in genetic engineering made fresh supplies of interferon a strong possibility and lent fuel to interferon's unprecendented explosion in the press, labs, and boardrooms of the past two years.

chapter 8

THE INTERFERON EXPLOSION

8

Many drugs undergo breakthroughs, but few have to survive the excitement and pressure of the kind of explosion that rocked interferon in the past three years. Interferon leapt from the backstage of quiet research into the gaudy spotlight of public exposure with a clamor that out-thundered any other biological event of the decade. How this biological big bang occurred proved fascinating in its study of the varying roles of power politics, psychology, and pure science in developing research products today.

For some twenty years, interferon struggled in the backwaters of scientific inquiry. It was difficult to use, difficult to identify, and troublesome to explain. It didn't seem to have any serious role in treating human disease. It was a washout, a scientific curiosity that had never lived up to its brief, early promise.

But in the past couple of years a remarkable confluence of capability, circumstance, and conjecture has swelled interest concerning interferon to flashflood proportions. From almost total anonymity, the protein has been elevated to the pedestal of myth and mystery.

Suddenly, interferon has become the stuff of fan magazines and gossip columns. When John Wayne was fading toward his last sunset, what miracle drug did doctors consider trying in a last ditch effort to corral his cancer? Interferon. In the Shah of Iran's final days, what substance stood at the center of veiled transactions between Europe and Egypt? Interferon. Rumors like this helped enflame passionate speculation about the drug, scarcely diminished by the fact that both famed pseudo-recipients died.

With a public bombarded by reports of weird cancer treatments—laetrile, vitamins, hot oil baths, mental power—the mere fact that interferon did not draw the same total annihilating scorn from sober scientists came to be seen as de facto proof that it *must work*. Every time a publication asked "Can Interferon Cure Cancer?" thousands assumed that the answer must be yes, or no one would dare hazard asking the question in public.

The situation that arose was bad for everyone involved. Patients, scientists, and research funders all paid a heavy price for interferon's lunge to prominence. And the drug itself suffered most of all. The overblown, unrealistic, confused picture of it that emerged made it hard for any of interferon's bona fide abilities to receive the exposure they deserved.

Problems didn't stem from the fact that interferon didn't work. In fact, it was demonstrating startling abilities against cancer tumors, and it also had unmatched clout against all sorts of viruses. The protein promised to become a major tool for physicians in the 1980s and 1990s.

But it wasn't God's own elixir! It didn't cure everything. The reality was that scientists hadn't—and still haven't—been able to test it thoroughly enough to know exactly what it can or what it can't do.

As a result, disappointments can't be avoided. They have an inevitability about them that nobody's good intentions can deflect. For better or for worse—usually for worse—they must struggle against a tide of inflated expectations.

In the beginning, there was skepticism. Even as late as 1975, when Mathilde Krim held her pivotal international symposium on interferon, the preponderance of scientific opinion was to wait and see if any of the zealots came up with something really big. Hans Strander's results were pooh-poohed because he had not been careful enough to include a statistically valid control group. Everyone was glad that he was getting good survival rates, but many felt he had done little to prove that interferon had anything to do with it.

Others felt that the seed of promise was there, but other possibilities should get higher priorities, since there wasn't enough interferon around to treat anyone, even if it had worked. Among the supporters of the protein were well-connected zealots chafing with impatience at the thought that a substance of such promise was going to be allowed to languish in the scientific hinterlands.

Chief among them in America was Krim, who found the skepticism she faced in the mid-seventies unfathomable and infuriating:

"Whether the skepticism is founded or not is a matter of opinion.

Perhaps in some cases one can say that it resulted from ignorance, lack of imagination and lack of reason rather than being unfounded. That was my opinion. I felt at least ten years ago there was ample justification for producing human interferon and testing it in man.

"Drug companies are not prepared to make investments without proof. Bureaucrats tend to be timid. They find it difficult to gamble with large amounts of money because they have to answer to the public. The difficulty of experimentation justified the reluctance of industry to invest; and the timidity of government altogether resulted in delaying for nineteen years developments that are necessary."

Other equally dedicated scientists felt, however, that there simply was not enough solid information about interferon yet available to justify raising the flag of hope and spending a pot of money. Dr. Frank Rauscher of the American Cancer Society was a confirmed skeptic about interferon and felt that going slowly in examining the new drug was eminently wise.

"In 1975, NCI began getting information from Sweden on Strander's work. I sent a team over there at that time to take a look at the data. My advisors came back, and they and I were both convinced that the data were not yet definitive enough to commit a large portion of the research dollars we had at that time to the program. So instead we committed about a half-million to production in this country for research purposes not clinical. I think it was a wise decision at that time. I was probably known as one of the most negative people in the country—maybe cautious. But, it is very important to use the public's funds as well as one can.

"The situation changed because of the work of Cantell and Strander and then because Cantell began making some of his interferon available for use in this country. We began getting anecdotal information, and became aware of the potential.

"It seemed to me that the time had come to bite the proverbial bullet." Rauscher sought "under conditions of controlled clinical trials that would be acceptable all over the world, to find out whether this material was as effective as some people thought it was."

The result was a simple press release that reverberated through the halls of research:

> *The American Cancer Society announced today that it plans to spend up to two million*

> *dollars for clinical testing to determine the possible value of human leukocyte interferon in the treatment of advanced cancer. Interferon is a natural body substance which has been shown to reduce the size of tumors in animal experiments as well as in a few scattered applications to human cancer patients. Its ultimate usefulness against cancer has yet to be proved.*[1]

Of all the potential cancer treatments it could have chosen to focus on, why did the Cancer Society select interferon?

For an explosion like interferon's to take place, a number of vital elements must be present and primed. Interferon had the fortune—it can be debated whether it was good, bad, or a combination—to reach a crucial point just when all these external factors were swelling to their limits.

A *Demand* In order for a scientific development to have explosive possibilities, a market must exist for its use. The bigger the market, the more sudden its emergence, the greater the explosion. The vast range of interferon's potential activities provided an unbelievable number of possible users, but the unpredictably fast ascendence of genetic engineering brought with it the potential for interferon to fulfill its promise in this decade. Truly, need is both apparent and extensive; with its sudden possibility, it is explosive.

Let's see how the thoughts of people in related fields can affect scientific developments. In Switzerland, Charles Weissmann was not an interferon researcher. He wasn't fascinated by viruses or cancer problems. He was enamored of genes and of the possibilities for enormous profit to be gained by tinkering with them.

He realized very soon that by molecular engineering it would be possible to produce very interesting chemicals in bacteria. Then he started thinking about which ones would be most interesting. The first one that came to mind was insulin, and he figured out on paper how to make it cheaply. There was a big industry which thrived on making insulin, but he figured you could muscle into this market by making it even cheaper. However, he found out that the potential difference was only a matter of a few percent. There was no point in making insulin bacteria; other people were doing that effectively. The next possibility was growth hormone. He said, "We can do that.

It will be feasible, but what is the market for growth hormone? We can only sell five micrograms over the next ten years." So then, he determined that he needed something that "cannot be produced economically in any other fashion, and which is active in small quantities because even with bacteria the amount of pure material that you get is small once it has passed through all these purification steps."

And so, he thought, interferon might be a good choice. It could not be manufactured economically in large enough quantities, and so its market was essentially free from competition. He went with his idea to the big pharmaceutical companies in Switzerland, but they weren't interested. So, he started his own company. This decision helped set the stage for interferon's catching fire.

Not only must a market need be present, but a mental need is necessary as well. An explosion is far more likely when funding agencies and the public are hungry for the type of discovery that is approaching realization. A discovery that doesn't touch a raw nerve in the public imagination will never explode; it may be terribly important and win Nobel prizes, but it won't explode.

Interferon came into the cancer research picture a godsend. Progress had been steady against malignancies for more than a decade, but it had also been extremely dull. The public was turned off by the kinds of advances science was coming up with. Scientific advances weren't catching people's attention, and they became burdened with so many limitations and such despicable side effects that no one could get enthusiastic about them, even if they helped keep patients alive a bit longer.

The time was ripe for a dramatic, provocative leap forward in cancer research—something totally different for the cancer establishment to use as a counterweight to laetrile and the other specious cures. Interferon clicked.

As Mathilde Krim explains, "the American Cancer Society and some of the others felt that they really would like to have something dramatic happen. They felt they were making progress but it wasn't dramatic enough—not enough progress to satisfy the public. They saw chemotherapy and felt that was not what they had expected to come out of all this. They wanted something that went whammo against cancer. I want something whammo against cancer too. The reality is that we couldn't get it then or now, and we have to be very happy with what we have. The desire, however, played a major role in spurring interferon. But that's not a criticism, you know. Everybody was very justified in wanting something whammo. I mean, some people think it's chic not to want to treat cancer normally. Interferon isn't scientifically acceptable, but has some of the advantages of the popular nontreatments like laetrile. It was exciting, mysterious."[2]

To a small extent, the exposure of scientifically unfounded cancer treatments, such as laetrile, hurt interferon's development. So many researchers and backers of treatment programs had been burned by the persistent notoriety of these quack procedures that they had grown incredibly calloused to any new, different approach.

As an anti-tumor agent, interferon was clearly new and bizarre. Its effects were completely different from any ever found before. So, in knee-jerk fashion, several conservative scientists attacked the anti-tumor findings in animals. They believed proponents were jumping to conclusions, and that though proponents were actually seeing an anti-viral effect in the lab animals, they were deluding themselves into thinking it had an anti-cancer potential. It seemed just another cancer hype.

There was, however, a significant difference between interferon and other novel approaches to cancer treatment. The people supporting it weren't fringe scientists; they didn't run clandestine clinics in Mexico. They were respected, solidly-credentialed researchers who were performing work under the strict rules of establishment science. Eventually, the weight of their reputations and collective evidence overcame the negative association of interferon's newness.

In part, this was aided by changes in thinking about how the body works and how cancer makes it go awry. In this mode, interferon supporters weren't speaking in opposition to existing ideas, but in complement to them. Mathilde Krim explains: "There has been a school of thought developing over the last ten or fifteen years that believes our body's immune system responds to the presence of tumors. It has been found that a number of substances can increase immunal activity and immune effectiveness. However, we can raise the possibility that this may not be quite right. It may not be the immune system that responds to the tumor, but the interferon system. It stimulates the immune response; it is in charge.

"Others might not agree with us. But the concept that there is a biological response to the presence of tumors, and a natural internal defense against them has been accepted. So, the idea of having a biological substance such as interferon having an effect on cancer cells is less weird today than it used to be."

At the moment when these concepts were becoming accepted widely among scientists, interferon began to show some real muscle in lab tests. It was felt, in many quarters, that this potential trigger of the bodily defenses should be tested quickly. If it worked, it would not only provide a worthwhile potential treatment, but would confirm the whole mode of thinking about the body's complicated interior protection capabilities. It could set off a research gold rush to find other substances and systems that could accomplish similar protections in different circumstances.

Arrayed against this growing feeling were entrenched ideas and jealousies among researchers in the cancer treatment and anti-viral fields. The cancer workers felt threatened at the looming presence of a treatment that could not only decrease the importance of existing methods, but could divert research attention and money into the entirely new field of biological control. Cancer chemists and radiologists wanted to hold up interferon to protect the primacy of their own methods. Not all of them reacted this way, but there certainly were a few who wielded considerable clout.

"You have to consider the psychology of the people who are doing the research on interferon in cancer," one immunopharmacologist has said. "They're immunotherapists. Immunotherapists have been working in the past with materials like BCG, a bacillus that's used as a general stimulus to the immune system of a cancer patient. BCG has a very limited effect. Other immunologic materials are even weaker—none of them make tumors shrink or cause partial regressions of disease.

"Along comes interferon, and behold—some tumors in some patients do shrink, and the immunologists get all excited. Compared to what they've been able to accomplish in the past, interferon looks pretty darn good.

"The critics of interferon, of course, are often oncologists who've been working with the highly toxic but sometimes very effective cytotoxic (cell-killing) drugs used in chemotherapy.

"To them, interferon is pretty thin stuff. They've seen big tumors dwindle down dramatically with chemotherapy. Not always, but it does happen. Chemotherapy is curing acute leukemia in children, it prevents the recurrence of bone cancer in 80 percent of patients, and with radiation therapy, it has made Hodgkin's disease almost totally curable. Naturally, they're going to be skeptical about interferon, because of where they're coming from, just as the immunologists are naturally going to be enthusiastic about it because of where they're coming from."[3]

As for the viral workers, they saw interferon as a virus medication and they wanted to keep it as a virus medication. They realized that if an anti-cancer potential were shown, their virus work would be forced to take a back seat in terms of money and importance to interferon cancer research. So they argued against pushing the drug forward.

"All these people were pushing their own attitudes, protecting their own turfs," states Mathilde Krim. "It was ridiculous."

And again, while jealous opposition slowed the expansion of interferon a bit, the weight of evidence and breadth of support had reached a point by 1978 where the protein couldn't be denied its share of research attention.

Cancer research needed an interferon to perk up public interest and keep up funding levels that benefitted all programs. Despite all doubts and disagreements, interferon was hustled to the head of the line.

Public Relations When a sense of impending explosion fills the air, everybody wants to get some mileage out of the boom. When interferon broke into the public arena, the explosiveness and novelty of its appearance fueled a self-propelling phenomenon that increased its importance.

Shell Oil, for instance, matched the American Cancer Society's $2 million offer amid a panoply of press attention. Now the people at Shell are certainly sincere in their desire to use some of their oil money to help researchers into a cure for cancer. They weren't in any way, shape, or form being socially derelict.

But, honestly, they picked interferon to give their money to because they knew it would get their name in all the papers. They knew that all those positive stories about how a big oil company cares about unfortunate folks with cancer would help offset some of the negative clout oil giants had gotten in the press.

The end result here isn't a bad thing—more money for interferon research—but it does tend to overblow the importance of the drug, for purposes other than scientific ones. Like the mute in Carson McCuller's *The Heart Is A Lonely Hunter,* a discovery on the verge of explosion is interpreted and used by everyone to his own end, often resulting in the confusion and despair of those closest to the source.

A Big Impediment The impediments to interferon research seemed to stifle the explosion; in actuality, they made it all the more powerful. The larger the problems, the greater the boom when they are overcome. The odds against getting men on the moon were so great they gave the accomplishment added weight in the public's eye. The incredible scarcity and cost of interferon meant that it couldn't follow a simple step–by–step development. Positive results, like water behind a dam, had to build up until the pressure for action was overwhelming. Only unbelievable pressure could generate the vast amounts of money required to support a barely decent level of interferon work. So, you have a situation where the costs are great, the risks high, and the pressure building to a peak of unrelenting intensity. These are the raw materials of explosion, and, in interferon's case, they produced a classic detonation of attention, funding, and anticipation.

Ability At the core of the explosion, of course, must lie the value of the discovery itself from a purely scientific point of view. It must be an ability that opens up new avenues. It must be practically as well as theoretically possible—postulating rings for Saturn doesn't cause an explosion, finding them does. It must have the potential for touching many lives, and must synthesize new modes of thought. Interferon qualified on all counts. No one could hope for a substance that hinted of being able to do more wonderful things.

The result of all these elements congregating around a discovery is the kind of worldwide mini-hysteria that swept interferon during 1978 and 1979. And sudden developments like that bring up an interesting "chicken-and-egg question." Which came first, the expansion of interest, or the importance? Which came first, increased interest in interferon, or increased amounts of interferon? Some scientists insist that the slight increase in interferon supplies brought about findings which in turn created the explosion. This in turn *really* picked up the interest in making and working on the protein. Others state, equally forcefully, that the findings created the explosion, and it was the expectation of the explosion that spurred increases in production, which have since been vastly magnified.

It's impossible to answer this riddle, but it points out how convoluted and interdependent the elements of a major scientific breakthrough can be.

Whatever the underpinnings and motive forces, the results of the 1978 interferon explosion are as clear as the crystal used to make lab glass. Suddenly, every biochemical outfit in the world jumped into interferon production. Genetic engineering might be the ultimate production method for the protein, but it could be years off. In the meantime, a lot of testing was going to be done and everybody wanted to get some of that business. After twenty years alone in his lab, Kari Cantell would have an instant assemblage of competitors, something he had been hoping would happen for years.

Staid pharmaceutical firms, such as Calbiochem-Behring, a division of American Hoechst, began putting Cantell's system to work on a massive scale, while at MIT an entirely new method of production sprang into use.

Housed in a converted candy factory, the MIT interferon lab perfected the system of suspending interferon-producing cells from microscopic beads. This is a vast improvement over Cantell's system because it eliminates much of the handling required to produce interferon and opens the process to many other kinds of cells than leukocytes.

The cells are given a negative charge and the beads a positive one, keeping the pair clinging together while the cell grows and produces its interferon. In a comparison study between this method and the old one, MIT's technique produced ten to thirty times as much interferon per liter of cultured cells. The process has been hailed as a significant advance that could substantially and immediately lower interferon costs, while genetic engineering is working the kinks through its system.

Government, too, raised its ante on interferon. The National Cancer Institute talked Congress into a $13.5 million program studying "biological response modifiers." First on the list: interferon.

Around the world, interferon became an overnight priority:

> *Lyon, France:* Institut Merieux, the pharmaceutical division of the Rhone-Poulenc group, announced in June, 1980, that it would soon

be able to manufacture interferon on an industrial scale. A company official claimed they would be able to achieve better results than Kari Cantell's lab within one year.

Johannesburg, South Africa: The National Institute for Virology proclaimed in mid-1980 that South Africa would reach interferon production levels in early 1981 that would allow for the treatment of more than 3600 people. This would make South Africa the world's leading producer of leukocyte interferon.

Taipei, Taiwan: A joint project of the Taiwan government and the American Bureau for Medical Advancement in China announced plans to establish a leukocyte interferon facility in Taipei. Dr. David Habif of Columbia, one of the American Cancer Society interferon testers, is behind the project, and claimed production would start during 1981.

Belgrade, Yugoslavia: The Yugoslav Academy of Science's Institute of Immunology signed an agreement to sell interferon to National Patent Development Corporation of Brunswick, New Jersey to help get the American firm's interferon production program off the ground. National Patent will market the interferon the Slavs supply, in addition to manufacturing its own.

Meanwhile, in the USA:

G. D. Searle & Company, Chicago increases interferon involvement tenfold, including establishing a new plant for the protein's production in England.

Flow Laboratories, McLean, Virginia nets a $2 million National Cancer Institute contract

> to produce fibroblast interferon using the MIT method. Warner-Lambert gets $895 thousand for NCI leukocyte interferon production.
>
> Mathilde Krim and Sloan-Kettering get permission to set up a leukocyte interferon production facility in Switzerland. She believes it will match Cantell's production levels during the first year.
>
> The American Cancer Society weighing back into the maelstrom it spawned, antes up another $3.8 million, on top of the $2 million that started it all.

If the early lobbyists and the American Cancer Society were intent on luring business and government into the interferon fray, then they sure did a good job. And while this end result is gladdening, it must be said that interferon's explosion left much negative debris as well.

The intense press scrutiny of the drug and its proponents, the pressure for information and speculation, the intense desire of cancer patients for interferon created a cloud of confusion around the protein that may have actually slowed its acceptance by the scientific community.

And the dust from the blow-up left a bad taste in some people's mouths. Nicholas Von Hoffman thundered in the *Washington Post* that uncertainty about interferon's abilities "didn't discourage any number of persons in white smocks from making their debuts before the cameras to conjure up rose-hued dreams of therapeutic miracles. Not that they didn't say that things were still rather iffy, but that part got said rather quickly.

"Thousands of people must have been led to believe a cancer cure had been found. Such a discovery is a matter of only academic interest unless you have the disease or a loved one does. Then the truth is heartbreaking. This careless and unthinking public presentation of the possibilities of interferon must have broken the hope and hearts of a lot of people who didn't need to have their sadness and pain compounded by men and women of science who should know better."

Hoffman, in fairness, might just as well have attacked the men and women with notebooks who stood on the other end of these exchanges and carried the message of hype to the public. None of this grew from feelings of maliciousness or greed. Well-meaning people were simply reacting as best they could to extraordinary pressures. Their performance was not perfect. But then, who could have expected them to be?

chapter 9

INTERFERON AND THE GENETIC ENGINEERS

9

The predictions of genetic engineers provided the spark which detonated the current interferon explosion. Its next success depends largely upon them. They must create the vast new supply of the protein they promised. And then provide it in a form that people can use safely and effectively. They must prove that the potential of their new age technology can be translated into a widespread, practical product.

The odds for their success are very strong. In fact, clear signs of their impending transformation of the interferon sector—and much of biology—have already appeared.

One of the first came on January 16, 1980, when Charles Weissmann, a geneticist from the University of Zurich, and Walter Gilbert, a sharp-featured Harvard biologist, called a most unique press conference in the Boston Park Plaza Hotel. The gathering was striking for a number of reasons, not the least of which was the news the pair delivered: Weissmann had cloned and gotten expression of human leukocyte interferon in a biologically active form through recombinant DNA technology.

This was certainly major news, even though a Japanese team had already cloned fibroblast interferon in a biologically inactive state. What was perhaps even more arresting about the announcement, however, was that it wasn't sponsored by either professor's university, but by a corporation—Biogen, SA—set up to manufacture and profit from the new technology commonly called genetic engineering.

The press conference represented a break with the past in two completely different arenas. In science, it marked the moment in which genetic engineering moved from the shadowy world of lab studies to the front pages, and interferon moved from long-range scarcity to short-term abundance. In business, it denoted the first public appearance of the potentially enormous bioresearch industry, which could become as intertwined with our future medical care and pocketbooks as today's computer and electronics industries.

When Weissmann and Gilbert made their announcement in a hotel ballroom rather than in the pages of a staid scientific journal, and when they did it in the guise of incipient entrepreneurs rather than as non-involved researchers, they cast aside generations of scientific tradition. Not only did their announcement proclaim that it was a new day scientifically, but that it was a new age in the way scientists went about their business and used the knowledge they discovered.

Many cynics felt that the pair had made their presentation to the press instead of to other scientists not for the good of the public, but to enhance the reputation and worth of the company they had helped set up to exploit their findings. It is intriguing that one important science journal reviewed the conference with a comment not by a scientist, but by Scott King of the Wall Street analyst firm of F. Eberstadt and Company, who said the Biogen announcement "should not be interpreted to mean that it has any significant advantage in either technology or patent protection. Achieving expression of the (interferon) gene is only the first of many steps required to demonstrate a commercial process."

Exactly. As both Weissmann and Gilbert were scrupulous to emphasize at the conference, they were merely pointing up the potential of their discovery, not its immediate practical value. They had made an exciting—but not the ultimate—step forward.

Still, the media exploitation of the event led to much notoriety, public overexcitement, and misunderstanding which left many scientists grumpy and, frankly, envious. It was, to make an understatement, a rough way to begin a new age of research.

It was fitting that the first major announcement of the genetic engineering era should focus upon interferon. The two developments have been closely intertwined since both rose to prominence among scientists in the 1970s.

The possibilities of genetic engineering lay behind the timing and size of interferon's explosion into the eighties. Their fates were inherently linked. If either proved a spectacular failure, the other would suffer enormously. But if both proved true to their early indications, they would open an entirely new realm of science and blast into the financial stratosphere a seminal new business.

The importance to science of what Weissmann and Gilbert had to say that day must be carefully weighed. Clearly, they had made a breakthrough, but just as clearly they had failed to clear up innumerable problems that could render their process worthless long before it hit the market. William Stewart of Sloan-Kettering's Interferon Evaluation Program cautiously admitted that Weissmann's process could prove better than existing methods of making interferon. On the other hand, the product might prove useless in humans for many different reasons. And Thomas Merigan from Stanford said the process showed "hope" for the future, but was still far inferior to Kari Cantell's old, reliable production facility in Finland.

The tide of the future was becoming clear long before the controversial press conference, however. Molecular genetics was on the threshold of public and scientific acceptance, and whatever its problems and limitations, the emerging techniques of genetic engineering were clearly the wave of tomorrow.

"We're close to being able to know just about anything we want to know about molecular genetics," says Nobel Laureate David Baltimore of Massachusetts Institute of Technology. "I know that's an audacious statement. But we're at the point now that if we know how to ask the questions, the methods are there to answer it—although it may take years or decades."

"Thus in the forseeable future, we will understand cancer, genetic disease, aging, and the development and function of the nervous system."

By January 1980, scientists had reached the point where they had all the tools they needed to work their genetic magic. A mouse had been successfully cloned. They no longer needed to figure out what to do, merely how to do it more efficiently. They knew genetic engineering could work. They knew they could use bacteria and other forms of life to produce a cornucopia of chemicals with applications in every facet of research, business and common life. But they still didn't know if any of the chemicals they produced would be as worthwhile as their studies, equations and hopes told them they would be.

And their predictions glowed with promise. Scott King, the financial analyst, studied the field and stated unequivocally that by 1985 interferon produced through genetic engineering would be approved by the federal Food and Drug Administration for use in humans. Another business analyst predicted that within two or three years, interferon will be "very broadly" available for cancer treatment and ubiquitous for viral treatments a year later. And the cost per dose, he said, will plummet from fifty to two dollars. Almost universally, even the most optimistic pronouncements were followed by the caveat "and it could go even faster than that, and with good reason." For instance, in September 1979, reports to a recombinant DNA conference concluded that human interferon production was at least three years down the road. The shocking press conference followed a mere four months later.

But what about the usefulness of material produced by this strange new technique? At the time of the press conference no one, not even the researchers, was sure whether the interferon would work in people. However, in mid-1980 at a conference in Washington, another newly-sprouted genetic engineering company, Genentech, announced that it had produced four different strains of leukocyte interferon through cloning, and had given doses to spider monkeys exposed to a virus. The interferon treatment began just before infection and continued for seventy-two hours afterward. Three monkeys who received the artificial interferon did not develop infections. Three monkeys who received nothing contracted the virus. So, preliminarily at least, the genetically engineered interferon seemed to work like the real thing against viruses.

Such deeply significant findings are amazing considering that eight years ago California scientists, following in the footsteps of the genetic research of James Watson and Frances Crick, figured out the rudiments of the system to create living factories that produce chemicals on command. Even from the first moment, the scientists involved realized that they had on their hands a process that made any other biological production system seem archaic. In time they realized recombinant DNA could transform biology as the transistor transformed electronics.

The techniques behind this revolution are relatively simple. Scientists have found that some strands of DNA, the material that comprises our genes, are twisted into rings called *plasmids*. Certain enzymes can snip genes from these plasmids, and other enzymes can fuse new gene material into the breach. The added gene becomes part of the cell's genetic information, which controls what it does and how it lives. Most experiments to date have been done with an organism found in the human colon called *E. coli*.

If the new gene tells the *E. coli* to make a protein it has never made before, it will. If it commands the microbe to produce a deadly poison, it will. The body has no control over the action of its genes; they are in charge. So, by inserting the right ones, scientists can make the body produce whatever they want it to.

If interferon were the only potential product of genetic engineering, the technique would certainly not be the center of attention it is today. And, concurrently, the prospects for interferon's widespread availability and use would not be nearly as bright. But, fortunately, genetic engineering holds hope for being one of the most widely useful scientific processes ever discovered. The prospects are very exciting for researchers, business leaders, and writers. As an article in *Newsweek* wondered:

"How big is the market for a process that makes plants manufacture their own fertilizer? For microorganisms that mine silver, gold and copper ore? For chemicals that could be used for everything from floor wax to salad dressing? The answers are impossible to calculate with any precision, but by every estimate, the possibilities for the infant industry spawned by molecular biology are staggering. 'This work is broader in importance than anything since the discovery of atomic particles,' says Irving S. Johnson, vice president for research at Eli Lilly and Co. 'The commercial applications for recombinant DNA are limited only to the imaginations of the people using it.' "[1]

Genetic engineering looks like it will be able to produce a virtually limitless number of chemicals faster and cheaper than present methods. "You can take the DNA from a conventional antibiotic-producing strain of microorganism which normally grows very slowly," says J. Leslie Glick, head of the small biotechnology firm Genex, "and stick it into a fast growing microorganism to produce a good deal of that antibiotic in a much shorter time." High quality, low cost, constant production. It's a mercantile dream and a scientific tool of awesome potency.

Among the areas that this new technology will touch are:

Energy. Genetically engineered bacteria can generate lubricants, and possibly even organic fuels. They can also work to distill grains for incredibly cheap gasohol. National Distillers and Chemical Corporation, which makes Almaden wines and Old Grand Dad whiskey, has applied for patents in genetic alcohol production. Imagine, too, an organism that could leach the oil from shale and tar and sand without the energy profligacy and pollution of extraction plants.

Medicine. E. F. Hutton has declared that production of human insulin will be "one of the first major product battlegrounds" of genetic engineering. The allure here is the huge number of people who need the drug and who could benefit from a cheaper supply. Endorphin, the brain's natural pain fighter, has been successfully produced through recombinant DNA, too. The wide availability of this chemical and the possibility of implanting the endorphin production command in cells could revolutionize painkilling techniques. Man-made organisms will also be involved in producing human growth hormone that will alleviate problems for dwarves and an uncountable range of enzymes, hormones and other organic chemicals for use in medications and research.

Chemistry. Experts have estimated that widespread application of genetic engineering to chemical production could reduce the industry's huge energy requirements by 30 to 50 percent. Genetically engineered beasties could produce the raw material for plastics, antifreezes, alcohols, amines and dozens of other manufacturing substances. Cetus, a recombinant DNA firm, and Standard Oil of California plan to build a $15 million plant to produce some 400 million pounds of genetically engineered industrial chemicals per year.

Agriculture and Livestock. How about four season fruits that withstand frost? Or, consider the impact of genetically produced fertilizers that require no petroleum or expensive processing. Go a step further and think about crops that bind their own nitrogen, doing away with the need for fertilizer altogether. Recombined bug might even be crafted to generate edible material. Then there is the thought of supercows, ducks and horses, bred from cells genetically engineered for optimum performance characteristics.

The growth of the new genetic engineering industry is spearheaded by a cadre of small, entrepreneurial, aggressive, fiercely competitive companies. Most of them were started by or with scientists who realized this process was not the typical lab curiosity. Now they are clawing forward at breakneck speed, each trying to be first to the market where unbelievable profits await.

The business is unique because it sprang up without outside inducement. It was a seemingly unplanned program put together by unconnected sets of experts. A ragtag brigade of scientists, investors, and managers generated a potentially major American industry with incredible speed and spontaneity.

The ambitions of the companies thus created are fittingly bold. "Our goal is to be a fully-integrated, complete corporation," says Robert F. Byrnes, vice-president for marketing at Genentech. Robert Cawthorn, Biogen's president, trumpets that: "We plan to become a large commercial company on the basis of recombinant DNA technology, not just a contract research firm."

The industry's elder stateman is Cetus Corporation, created in 1971 by Dr. Peter Farley, now its president, and Ronald E. Cape, now chairman. They were convinced that fortunes could be made in biology, just as they had been in other branches of science. Cape states: "There had been a couple of dozen Nobel prizes for the discovery of the secrets of life, yet when you looked around for a practical application there wasn't a single one." His company was going to establish some. They managed to fire up three other risk takers, including Don Glaser, a researcher who had won a Nobel prize in physics before turning to biology, to sign on.

Then the fledgling company went to the world's leading pharmaceutical firms insisting it could improve their best strains of antibiotic cell lines. And for those few willing to give them a chance they did. The company was audacious; it demanded huge royalties for its successes, and carried itself with a swagger which helped convince the bigshots that the upstarts knew what they were doing.

By 1976, Cetus had grown to seventy-five employees and began its long planned movement into the mainstream of lab business. It moved from pharmaceuticals into other areas of genetic production; it was on its way to becoming a widely divergent, full-service gene tinkerer.

Cetus, today, has big dreams. It expects to employ some 450 people by 1985, and to build up a stock value of more than $1 billion by the end of the decade. It has already acquired $12 million by selling company shares to Standard Oil of California, along with significant investments from Standard of Indiana and National Distillers.

Interferon plays a central role in the company's plans. It has committed twenty-eight employees, including thirteen Ph.D.s, to the project full-time, and has spent more than $5 million for three years of research, which it expects to double by 1983. Genetically engineered interferon could, says a company official, "be the largest, single most important medical development you and I will ever see."

Cetus is not shy about its goal of climbing to the top of the corporate heap. "We will be the biggest, run the fastest, and gather up the major opportunities," declares Peter J. Farley. But he admits there is still "plenty of room for everyone. I think the industry will be massive; it cuts across artificial lines of demarcation among chemistry, food, agriculture, and energy. We'll be around fifty years from now as a major corporation."

Another early entrant into the field was Genentech, formed by a small band of scientific entrepreneurs in south San Francisco. The movers behind the company, created in 1976, were Dr. Robert Swanson and Dr. Herb Boyer who saw recombinant DNA as a medical manufacturing marvel far before most other people. Only a year after the company got started, the team produced the first successfully engineered product, a brain hormone somatostatin. They had proved the new technology really worked, though the limited-use hormone didn't reap any financial prizes.

With that accomplished, the company's movers turned their sight toward insulin. In only ten months, they had created the medication in microbes. The breakthrough held enormous financial potential because three and a half million Americans require insulin, which they now must get from animals. Human insulin would be both cheaper, and most likely safer. Now, the product is undergoing testing for FDA approval, which should come in a year or two.

After insulin, Genentech went after human growth hormone, which it is now scaling into production capacity. And ahead looms interferon, to which the firm has assigned twelve researchers full-time.

"The technology is now moving very rapidly—more rapidly than I would have predicted," says Swanson. "The benefits that many people thought were five to ten years away are going to be here in two or three years. For instance, we're going to be testing our interferon in humans far sooner than anyone expected.

"The science started in the academic environment, but most academics aren't willing to put up with the bureaucracy of many large corporations. At Genentech, we provide an environment where there isn't a bureaucracy, where there's a lot of scientific freedom and the ability to pursue your own ideas as well as the ability to get some of these products out to the public."[2]

Genentech's interferon success is at the forefront of the industry. Company scientists have reported bacterial yields of interferon as high as 100,000 molecules per bacterial cell, far higher than the levels Weissman announced at his press conference. The company has gotten government approval to produce interferon batches as large as 600 liters, which would produce between twenty to forty milligrams of pure interferon per liter.

By late 1981, Genentech hopes to have enough interferon "to initiate clinical trials to assess and document the substance's safety and efficacy," in the words of a company officer.[3]

Such successes bring sky-high hopes. E.F. Hutton, for instance, considered conservative Genentech's belief that it will have 1,000 employees and revenues of $100 million by 1985.

Generally speaking, experts in the financial markets are extremely high on genetic engineering. E.F. Hutton's drug industry analyst Nelson Schneider stated that Weissmann's interferon announcement, "showed recombinant-DNA research had reached beyond the model-T stage." Another Wall Street analyst notes that interest in the field is almost fevered. "People really don't understand anything at all about this field," he states. "All they want to know is how to invest in it."

Recently, Genentech broke more new ground in the field by going public. The stock offering by the company caused a rampage on Wall Street, despite the fact that it has never paid a dividend and has no products in the marketplace. The incredible surge of the stock to almost triple the offering price was as much a ringing endorsement of the new direction in biology as a reasoned decision about this one company, which is still wrangling about whether it, or some of the universities who launched its scientists, holds full right to its discoveries.

Genex is a Maryland genetic engineering firm which grew from the quick thinking of its chairman Robert F. Johnson. "I was at the National Academy of Sciences Forum," he recalls. "I had an intuitive feeling that this area would be important, but the antagonisms shown at the meeting convinced me the big companies would be scared off."

So, he decided to fill the gap, hit the road for financing and eventually set up his own small recombinant lab. Unlike the flashier

West Coast companies, Genex plans to center its efforts on industrial chemicals rather than genetically engineered natural products. They want to avoid the long process of clinical trials and permissions these products will require. Industrial chemicals can be marketed more quickly. So, Genex probably won't be as hotly involved in the interferon sweepstakes as the other ground-floor firms.

Then, of course, there is Biogen, the Swiss company that broke the story in the newspapers. Biogen was set up by scientists because the big drug companies didn't seem interested in investing in genetic engineering research—at least not under their own names—since they feared the controversy and speculation swirling around the techniques. Shortly thereafter, however, the huge Schering-Plough Corporation bought a large chunk of Biogen stock and the right to develop its discoveries for the marketplace.

More forthrightly than other firms, Biogen has stated its intent to try to be first to the market with human interferon. And it has a first shot. Weissmann feels he can get his genetically engineered product up to marketable standards by sometime in 1981. It has already undergone a full range of lab tests, and has reacted just like human interferon in every one of them. "There is no way to exaggerate the importance of what's going on," Weissmann says. "This is a real revolution."

Just how Weissmann's small band of geneticists managed to achieve their interferon breakthrough explains a great deal about both how remarkable and how crude genetic engineering is today, and how elbow grease and the willingness to take risks still count for something in today's conservative business and scientific worlds.

Because of his discoveries, Weissmann is a rich man today, though mostly on paper. His wealth will grow more tangible, most likely, in a few short years, as will that of everyone else who got in on the ground floor at Biogen. That was part of the reason the company was set up in the beginning.

"As for the rewards," Weissmann says, "no, I haven't made any profit yet. It may be against the image of the scientist, but there's nothing wrong with making money."[4]

Weissmann's spanking clean, bright, modern research center in the suburbs of Zurich is a faithful indication of the financial possibilities of the field. But the disheveled casualness of the workers, and the frenetic pace of the work belie any image of capitalists resting on their laurels. With so much still to learn, there is hardly time for anyone to think about all those millions waiting to be had. So hectic was the pace at Weissmann's lab when the interferon breakthrough seemed close, that a bottle of champagne he'd bought for the occasion was forgotten; it wasn't opened until two months later.

Such fierce concentration was understandable considering the difficulty of working with interferon for recombinant DNA. Weissmann knew that if he could obtain an interferon gene and splice it into *E. coli*, he could generate some kind of interferon. His first problem was in trying to locate the gene. To do this, he needed to find *interferon-messenger-RNA*, the chemical instruction sheet that cells manufacture when invaded by viruses. It carries a negative image of the interferon working radical. If a geneticist can find the messenger-RNA, he can use it to determine the pattern of the gene that created it.

Interferon-RNA, however, was even harder to isolate than interferon itself. Imagine how scarce interferon is—mere molecules per cell which you can barely pick up through their action on the cell. But there is even less messenger-RNA, and its action is much harder to locate.

Weissmann decided to skirt the issue. Instead of trying to cull interferon-RNA from the mass of different messengers cells produce, he dumped RNA from some 20,000 genes encoded inside leukocyte cells, and decided to work with them all at once. Somewhere in there, he figured, there must be interferon-RNA. Instead of trying to extract the messenger, he would try to isolate interferon producing bacteria—that is, after the genetic splicing had been done.

So, he went through the plasmid snipping and splicing with all the RNAs he had collected. This is called the shotgun, or, in Walter Gilbert's phrase "the brute force" approach to recombinant DNA. All of the engineered *E. coli* was separated, a cell at a time, and cultured in the lab. Each culture carried the genetic messengers of one cell.

After sufficient time for growth had passed, the cultures were tested for the presence of interferon in an experiment much like the original discovery test. Cultures that were not making the protein were eliminated. Those that were, some 20,000, were placed into groups of 512, each split into eight units of sixty-four cultures. Each of these was tested, and again the successful group was subdivided and retested. After eighteen months of painstaking study and testing, Weissmann narrowed the field down to one supreme producing culture. It was in culture 2H, tray *Lambda*-8. It produced more active interferon than any of the other 20,000 tries.

"I don't consider my experiment a major scientific achievement," Weissmann says, "but I'd say it was a showpiece example of this kind of work. I've done more elegant work in the past, but no experiment gave me such a real sense of delight.

"Things are moving along in a pleasant way. Already we've improved the strain of bacteria to where it's producing twenty times more interferon than originally. It's clear now that the process will be commercially feasible."

Although Weissmann's first manufactured *E. coli* clearly produced interferon that was biologically active, they didn't make much of it. The amounts of interferon produced were actually lower than the levels achieved by Kari Cantell in Finland. Over the winter, Weissmann worked to increase his yields to levels that would bring the price of his interferon down to a commercially attractive level.

This was done by a similarly involved method of finding the original interferon producing colony. Weissmann took the original interferon generator and split it into groups. The group with the highest production level was split again, and so on in a painstaking process to isolate the single colony, even the single *E. coli* cell best capable of generating interferon.

After that, Weissmann faced the problem of purification. Cantell's interferon can be used to treat humans even though it is as sloppy as can be because everything in it comes from humans. Genetically engineered interferon, however, is the product of a bacteria, not a human. So it comes under rules of purity far stricter than Cantell's soup. Weissmann will have to be able to produce 100 percent pure interferon before the health boards of major countries will let him sell it for use on people—even for tests.

No government will chance being the one to have a genetically engineered epidemic on its hands. Purity is essential. The monoclonal antibody recently isolated in England—which is explained more fully in an earlier chapter—will probably be the method for achieving the necessary level of safety. Since the antibody clings to no other substance than interferon, it assures that all the interferon can be lifted from any mixture. Once the antibody is stripped away, only the interferon is left, utterly pure. "Monoclonal antibodies offer a safeguard in purification that is not provided by other methods of purification," says Derek Burke, "because you use the unique power of the antibody to recognize a particular antigen to bring about a purification process that is absolute. Not only can you show it to be more effective, but it is theoretically less open to objections than any other method."

The accomplishment of all these steps will probably take much of 1981. Then the approval process will begin, and only after that will any widespread human trials with genetically engineered interferon take place. But the process already achieved by Weissmann and the other pioneers has set in motion a flywheel effect that is adding momentum to genetic engineering while the slow process of actualization continues. The scent of triumph in this field has drawn around all of the profit-hungry "johnny-come-latelies."

Among them are many of the huge pharmaceutical companies that had the earliest opportunity to develop the technology but didn't want to take the risk. It is easier and safer for big companies to invest quietly in small experimental companies when a drug gets underway, than to undertake programs themselves. If the drug works, they can always buy out one of the small firms; and if it fails, they won't have any public egg on their faces. The fear that interferon could shrivel into a high–powered laetrile—a sham treatment that left bitter feelings behind it—made them even more reticent to identify themselves with the drug in any way.

Now they are jumping aboard for defensive reasons. They worry that the new techniques will make many of their traditional products unmarketable. Some half-dozen of the industry's big shots, including Eli Lilly, Miles Laboratories, Merck, and others have begun programs of their own. And others like Schering-Plough, Standard Oil, Monsanto, and DuPont have signed contracts with or bought into the smaller, more innovative firms.

Other small companies already involved in biological technology are testing the genetic engineering waters, too. Bethesda Research Laboratories, a five-year-old biotech company, announced in March, 1980 that it had achieved cloning of a gene involved in production of proline, an important amino acid. New England BioLabs, a tiny company in Beverly, Massachusetts, has the honor of being the first company to bring a genetically engineered product to market, albeit a rather specialized one. It's an enzyme produced by DNA. A third company, Collaborative Genetics, is focusing on using genetic engineering with yeasts for various industrial uses.

Any and all of these firms, large and small, may play a role in the future of interferon. As knowledge in the field grows and the flywheel-effect intensifies, discoveries of all sorts will be announced. The experience gleaned in producimg interferon will aid development of other genetically engineered products, and advances elsewhere will certainly help the development of commercial, genetically engineered interferon. As the field's parameters are extended, interferon will be made more applicable and more available.

If the current rate of growth in genetic engineering is any indication, interferon's supply will come sooner and larger than most people expected. Labs are turning up everywhere. No one wants to miss out on what looks like the first major commercial application. A quick review shows the extent of the spread:

England—After considerable foot dragging, Britain's National Enterprise Board has decided to go ahead and form the country's first formal biotech company, Celltech. The initial budget for the firm will be between $25 and $36 million over the next four or five years, a small amount designed to keep the firm "lean and hungry" and on the prowl for profit making projects. The company hopes to emulate America's success stories in genetic engineering, without some of the more vicious cutthroat aspects of their commercial rivalry.

Holland—In 1975, the Netherlands had seven recombinant DNA projects. By the end of 1979 there were seventy-eight, ten of which were backed by industrial firms. The country's research facilities still aren't up to world standards, but work is progressing swiftly anyway as both actual developments and the field's safety record overcome long-standing public and government unease about tinkering with genes.

Japan—The first successful interferon cloning took place here, and the commercially-minded Japanese are continuing to press forward toward creation of recombinant products their extraordinary industrial system can exploit.

For all its promise and explosive growth, the field is not without its problems. One that has tremendous implications for the mass-production of interferon is the question of patenting new forms of life. In June, 1980, the United States Supreme Court ruled that General Electric was entitled to request a patent for its oil-eating bug—a microbe that could gobble oil slicks before they endanger beaches. Government prosecutors had argued that opening up patents to new forms of life raised 1984-ish questions about the possibility of owning another creature, conceivably, in time, an android.

But the court felt that the new genetically engineered products were truly inventions and so the engineers were entitled to the same protection as any other inventor. Prior to this decision, an enormous pressure had built up as discoveries were being made, patents requested—and all stacked up in government offices while the case was being argued.

When the decision came down, a plethora of patents rushed through the bureaucracy, including rights to interferon production processes. The ability to patent genetic engineering processes has several important impacts on interferon's production. First, without patent protection, all the small firms in genetic engineering are likely to remain highly secretive; they don't want anyone to understand their processes. This slows the dissemination of information and, consequently, impedes development.

More importantly, patents encourage companies to try besting each other's processes. In other words, if Weissmann's patented process creates interferon for, say, $4 a dose, Genentech and others can either license Weissmann's process and pay him a royalty, or come up with their own more efficient system. The competition to create and patent even better systems stimulates production and lowers costs.

On the other hand, some genetic engineering firms might decide to keep their processes secret despite the protection patents might bring. In the case of a company which has made a true breakthrough, the process itself may be almost unreproducible elsewhere. If the process remains secret, the company will have a virtual monopoly on the product produced. Receiving a patent means making the process public, and some firms may decide not to do this.

In any case, the Supreme Court decision allowing patents on cloned forms was a watershed moment in the development of both the technology and the interferon itself. It was a universal green light that society was prepared to accept the new technology and give its purveyors the same benefits and protection as other businesses. It was a huge shot-in-the-arm for the burgeoning business.

The most serious worry many scientists have about genetic engineering has nothing to do with the process itself. They worry, instead, about the way it is being developed. They fear that the sudden influx of riches and shifty-eyed commercialism into supposedly scientific research could warp it beyond recognition.

The undercurrent sprang up with the Biogen press conference. "Why," questioned Stanford University science writer, Spyros Andreopolos, in the *New England Journal of Medicine*, "didn't the researchers choose the accepted channels for their announcement? . . . . What I am concerned about is the trend that is being established: In place of published data, open to all for examination and critical review, we now get scientific information by press conference. The abrogation by scientists of the normal processes of scientific communication does not help science or the reporters covering it."[5]

Others with similar worries point out that the initial genetic engineering breakthroughs came during a lunch break at a biologists' conference. Scientists like to go off in the evenings and kick ideas around, the argument goes, and people who are being secretive won't participate and will suffer as a result.

Traditional research will also suffer because of the availability of business money. "There are millions of dollars floating around. If you claim you've done something fancy you can raise a lot of money," one noted molecular biologist said. "The question is what will this do to the academic atmosphere?" Already, Peter Seeburg has come under fire for taking vital experimental chemicals with him when he left the University of California at San Francisco for Genentech. He claimed they were part of his work; the university claimed he was crippling their research in favor of the commercial lure.

Some scientists wonder just how impartial a researcher can be when his discoveries could line his pockets with silver. "Just as war-related academic research compromised a generation of scientists, we must anticipate a similar demise in scientific integrity when corporate funds have an undue influence over academic research," contends Sheldon Krimsky of Tufts University, a member of the National Institutes of Health Recombinant DNA Advisory Committee.

Walter Bodmer, of Britain's Imperial Cancer Research Fund, worries that the sudden influx of megabucks into research could twist it in unfortunate directions:

"I think there is a danger because now the sort of scientists that are working in these areas have little background in commercial contacts, and all of a sudden, people who were studying some obscure bacterium and its genetics, find themselves able to do things that have financial value and are elevated to the commercial setting.

"So obviously there's a distortion in the evolution of the learning process. But chemists, physicists, and engineers have had these contacts and been involved in this for years. I think what's happening now is that biologists are getting into a situation that is probably quite familiar to other groups of scientists.

"I think it's a learning process, and I think there will be problems in the relationship between the academic and the commercial setting, and I think there will be lessons to be learned. We will just have to live with it. I think it will have a lot of advantages, such as a lot more jobs for people in these areas. But I think it has to be carefully watched, and there are bound to be some distortions."[6]

Derek Burke is concerned that the sudden shift toward commerce for development of scientific ideas will irreparably harm the vital training grounds of future scientists—universities:

"There are those in universities who perhaps are getting sucked into this commercial field. They instantly become much more competitive. But that's inevitable. As somebody said last week, it's like studying to hold up an express train. I'll just get crushed. We university scientists are just going to have to get out of these fields because we simply can't compete.

"I'm also rather discouraged about some of the attitudes in industry, which are unrealistic about what the universities can and can't do. They expect things from universities which universities are in no position to give. I think that we are running the system down and I'm not sure whether it'll be able to continue.

"In a university, the traditional way of doing this has been to employ young research fellows, who would work on their Ph.D. in a very productive phase of their careers for five or six years. Then they move on to another position and become more involved in management and their own projects. Now that's stopping because the system depends upon having jobs that these people go to. There are no new jobs for these people to go to; they're not coming into the system. They are going to industry."

The enormous potential for change was drastically demonstrated when Harvard University considered establishing its own company to exploit patents stemming from research by Harvard scientists. Harvard planned to hang on to a minority share in the company, spreading the largesse among scientists, management, and venture capital companies. In the past, Harvard was willing to let scientists develop projects with private companies. Harvard received royalties on any patents that resulted. Now, the shocking amounts involved spurred the college to re-think the situation. A bitter controversy resulted when the school's considerations were announced.

Could a university remain impartial in funding its research if some of the projects resulted in profits and others didn't? Could classics possibly compete for support when a university corporation is more enamoured with the financial productivity of microbes? Can an institution of learning sustain its primary role when buffeted by the pressures of competing with full-time corporations, or would the profit-making need subjugate educational ones, with Harvard U. becoming Harvard, Inc.?

Daniel Steiner, counsel to the university, wrote that, "When considering the promotion of a junior faculty member whose work might offer considerable commercial promise, the possibility of financial return must not prejudice or be seen to prejudice the academic decision on promotion. The possibility of compromise of the university's academic integrity is unavoidably present in a variety of contexts, be it admissions or faculty appointments."[7]

The fierce opposition caused Harvard to back off of the proposal, but the implication remained.

Behind all this is the largely unspoken fear that the big commercial build-up will bring on a backlash from a public fed up with overweening, monied science-entrepreneurs. Some older researchers point out that atomic scientists were supposed to reap a bonanza during the nuclear age, but the result was a savage public backlash against their field and one of the worst public images of any branch of science.

"When scientists get too powerful," one leader in virology states, "the public comes to expect too much. And when they don't get all they expect, they feel they are being manipulated and they turn off."

But others counter with arguments that biologists have been unworldly. Chemists have been living in the commercial world for fifty years and still do exciting research. And that physics and chemistry have had their golden age. This is the Golden Age of Biology."

Is it? Will interferon actually be the vehicle for ushering in a nascent era of biological wonderment? Possibly, but such high-blown expectations can be their own worst enemy. "The enormous publicity given to the commercial potential of recombinant DNA may be counterproductive because it is creating unreal expectations. I think there are potentialities in the technology, but based on my experience with other technologies, the gap between a laboratory process and reduction to commercial reality is going to take much longer than the impression created in the numerous articles about the subject," states Orin Friedman, president of Collaborative Genetics.

One possible dark lining in the silver cloud, at least as far as interferon is concerned, is the possibility that genetic engineering will be beaten to the marketplace or outperformed there by the old-fashioned, muddling production method called sequencing. This involves stretching a protein or other chemical, and "reading" snips of it using transcription chemicals. Once the entire chain of components has been read, it can be reproduced by lining up the constituent parts in vats and chemically stitching them together in the proper order.

Mathilde Krim explains how sequenced interferon could sneak up behind the ballyhooed recombinant entrant:

"Recombinant DNA has caught people's imagination, but what about the synthetic approach? Once you have the sequence of DNA, knowing the genetic code, you can reconstitute the amino acid sequence of a protein such as interferon. You can make it synthetically. Now the interferon chain is bigger than any other that has been made synthetically so far. It's 166 links instead of thirty or seven or whatever. But you can still break it into links and test each little bit separately. That could be very interesting because we may well find the pieces of the molecule control different aspects of its activities. We thus might be able to form an abbreviation of interferon that does the same thing, but will be far cheaper. Or if it does only one of the essential things, it would be useful. We could sort of have a recipe that this is the anti-viral interferon, and this is the anti-carrier and so on. It has the same promise as genetic engineering. It may in fact win because once you get on the right sequence, it may be cheaper to make interferon synthetically."

The parallel between the genetic engineering movement as a whole and its first big product, interferon, is striking. Both have incredible potential, but they have also been strapped by extraordinary buildup and controversy. Both are beset by doubts and uncertainties. And yet, in the end, both will almost certainly fulfill at least a large measure of their vaunted possibilities.

For interferon the ultimate hope is control of cancer, and for the genetic engineering movement the ultimate end is no less than creation of an improved human species.

Already, a team at UCLA has successfully transferred a gene from cells of one mouse to those of another. The transplanted gene then spread out among the hosts' cells, carrying its new genetic information. Another team created a mouse embryo that was a clone of its parent. Martin J. Cline, director of the test, sees human applications at least three years away. When the time comes, the possibilities for such a transfer include placing drug-resistant genes into the cells of cancer patients so they can withstand greater chemotherapy levels, and also placing correcting genes into those victims with sickle cell or other congenital disorders.

Wouldn't it be splendid, too, if it becomes possible to insert the genetic code for interferon production into the cells around a cancer tumor. The local, internally-produced interferon levels might be able to far exceed safe dosages given through shots. The transformed cells might be capable of complete resistance to malignancy, by surrounding the cancer mass and isolating it for maximum effective treatment. Could a patient's cells be removed, and then transformed genetically into a potent, permanent, interferon-based virus vaccine?

Possibly. Not certainly, not immediately, not unquestionably. But, definitely possible.

chapter 10

LOOKING FORWARD

10

Interferon has followed a "roller coaster" course to its present promising state. From lionization as the new penicillin for viruses, it fell to near scientific anonymity. Then, because of both internal progress in the field and many advances in related subjects, the protein was "dusted off" and given a second opportunity for scientific prominence.

What is the status of interferon today?

It is a virus-fighting agent of unmatched range but problematical power. It has shown itself potent against every virus that nature or man has thrown against it. But it has also displayed limitations that keep it from becoming the wide-ranging preventative once hoped for.

As an anti-tumor drug, interferon has displayed increasing exciting abilities against an ever-expanding array of tumors. It has caused complete remission in some tumors, such as nonmalignant papilloma, and has caused tumors of at least a half-dozen other cancers to shrink.

The scarcity of the drug, however, has kept tests so small and of such short duration that the conclusions drawn from them must be muted. The abilities shown by interferon against tumors are not conclusive; the most accurate way to put it would probably be to say that findings are highly suggestive. They suggest a substance that doesn't kill cancer so much as control it. And it is this notion, that a natural substance from our own bodies can somehow modify the behavior of raging cancer cells, which so excites researchers.

Enough research has been conducted for one to state, categorically, that interferon is not the wonder drug to kill *all* cancers. In fact, our understanding of the complexities of this insidious family of diseases has reached the point today where it has become clear that a magic bullet cannot exist. Only the full understanding of every facet of every human cell will unlock the secrets of cancer's origins. And only a complete ability to follow the interactions of our environment and control it with our most basic life components, our genetic materials, will allow anyone to block cancer before it takes root. There are many who feel such knowledge is the product of distant dreams and not a realistic component of our future.

Despite these limitations, interferon has demonstrated itself a useful tool in the treatment of a number of tenacious cancers.

"Interferon and other biological response modifiers will not replace traditional therapies, but will enhance them," Jordan Gutterman says.

A clear, comprehensive view of expectations for interferon comes from Mathilde Krim, a dynamo behind interferon's current push to the fore in research. She expostulates on interferon with a raw passion that brooks no disapproval. But she is not a fanatic. Even scientists who disagree with her views, or feel she is too free in her speculations, admit that Krim is a superb researcher and organizer who only argues for what she truly believes is justifiable by the evidence.

At her tiny desk on the eleventh floor of Sloan-Kettering's main lab building on Manhattan's Upper East Side, Krim earnestly expounds on her favorite topic:

"I don't claim that interferon will be the magic bullet for cancer. I don't know that there is such a thing, to tell you the truth. But what other substance, at so early a stage in its development, has shown so much promising activity against different—often highly-resistant—strains of cancer? And can anyone name another cancer therapy that has shown so few side effects—all of them apparently reversible?"

Still, she admits, "It's really difficult at this point to say how much better interferon has performed with humans than other available treatments. You see, with chemotherapy we have statistics on large numbers of patients. With interferon, the largest groups are ten, fifteen patients, so you can't talk about percentages; they would not be significant.

"The figures mentioned so far don't mean too much, yet people are taking them at face value. For example, in Dr. Gutterman's study, about 40 percent of the patients responded. Now, he should not have used that figure because since he did, we've been stuck with it.

"Then along came some further studies, which were done on ten patients each. They show 10 or 20 percent responses, which are just as meaningless statistically as the original 40 percent number. But they are thrown in our face anyway and rumors spring up that recent trials have been disappointing. But it's all totally meaningless. We're trying to find out what it means.

"All the dickering over percentages and disappointment is ridiculous. The only thing that matters is that interferon shows activity against cancer. We know that now. Nobody questions that.

"What we have to determine is the level of activity. We have to improve our knowledge of the dose, the length of treatment. And we have to improve the purity of the material we're working with."

Krim accepts the fact that many scientists, even some working in the field, still have serious doubts about just how effective interferon will prove to be. Personally, however, she feels as strongly as possible that interferon will stand in the ranks of medicine's most important tools within a few years.

"Remember," she states wryly, "the first patients treated with penicillin died. The situations are similar. The results in both cases come from biological rather than chemical reactions. Penicillin at first was given in low dosages in a very impure state and its effects were very transient. It's a miracle, in fact, that they were observed at all.

"There may be different opinions, but mine is that interferon will rank at least as high as chemotherapy and radiation as a cancer treatment. And the beauty is that it can be added to the others and provide benefits they can't. Each treatment can build on the others.

"The problem with surgery, for instance, is that it can only work when we can see the tumors to cut them out. Interferon works on cancer cells wherever they are, even if we can't see a tumor at the location yet. Interferon—like chemotherapy, but with fewer side effects—can attack metastases before we know they are there.

"The trouble with today's treatment is that we can do very little about getting rid of residual cancer cells once the primary tumor has been attacked. We hesitate to use chemotherapy or radiation when definite signs of cancer aren't present because of their enormous side effects. A recurrence can get a toehold before we go in and try to stop it. In the future, I think we should follow surgery with an interferon course of treatment which would strengthen the patient's defenses so he can get rid of his residual cancer cells before they can form colonies. I think it will significantly decrease the percentage of recurrence."

In a 1980 speech to an interferon conference, Krim stated her credo for the immediate future of the field she helped to create: "There is ample and urgent work to be done in the interferon field. Although we cannot tell, as yet, how far the road ahead can take us, it is a road which is now already marked."

Beyond cancer, the potent protein has shown hints of startling abilities in other areas of medicine. Immune responses that plague transplant recipients seem to be suppressed by properly applied interferon. Obesity and Down's Syndrome have been linked, loosely, to interferon. Plants make it to protect themselves and the inability of some people to make it in the face of certain viruses might hold the key to understanding many chronic conditions.

Interferon is a spectacularly active, promising drug. But it's still proving itself in the scientific boonies. The clout of genetic engineering and newly spawned scientific enthusiasm will finally bring it to the forefront in the next couple of years. Until that fight is over, no one can be certain just how much of interferon's prowess is ingrained, how much is wishful thinking, and how much is hype.

In order to put the future of interferon in proper perspective, we should first look back to the origins and trials of another wonder drug of its age—penicillin. Today it seems incredible that there were ever doubts or low spots in the struggle to life of a drug so obviously useful. But there were. Let's suppose it is 1940 and war has begun. A few scientists are touting the efficacy of their new medication, a kind of mold, as an aid to wounded troops in combat. They go before the governments and pharmaceutical companies pleading for support. Here, in the words of Sir Ernst Chain, is what happened:

> *When after the clear demonstration of the curative effects of penicillin in clinical infections, it came to the question of producing penicillin in quantities large enough to use it for the treatment of war wound infections, the pharmaceutical industry on both sides of the Atlantic showed little enthusiasm to embark, even with full Government support, on research, let alone a major project of penicillin production by fermentation, because the penicillin yields available at the beginning were much too low to envisage practical clinical use of this substance; furthermore the*

> *fermentations were conducted at that time (with) a technique which did not lend itself to scaling-up. The pharmaceutical industry had no experience in the fermentation field, and little or no knowledge of the techniques. Furthermore, the most famous chemists, both in academic laboratories and industry, were absolutely sure that they would be able to synthesize penicillin, an apparently simple molecule, in a matter of a few months, and opposed the biological production by fermentation with all their might. At that time the organic chemists dominated the pharmaceutical industry.*
>
> *Eventually a company actively engaged in submerged fermentation, but with little experience in the pharmaceutical field, solved the problem of the industrial production of penicillin by submerged fermentation, helped by American government and university microbiological and genetic laboratories in which the yields of penicillin were increased. The penicillin produced was a very expensive product indeed, but the production was considered well worth the high cost in view of the incalculably valuable biological properties of this material for the war effort, making possible an effective treatment of bacterial infections of war wounds.*[1]

Despite its rocky beginnings, penicillin has far exceeded the expectations anyone held for it at the time. Today, laboratory yields of penicillin are 150 times greater than they were during the war.

Doubts about production, and doubts about worth. Despite its enormous potential, it had extraordinary costs. Only it needed vast backing to get it off the ground. The parallels between the early days of penicillin and those of interferon are remarkable. If it hadn't been for the demands of the war, penicillin might have followed a twenty-five year course to prominence similar to that of interferon.

The point is that new discoveries in science aren't neat; they don't emerge clearly and cleanly to universal acclaim. More often, they grow up slowly, surrounded by scorn from the short-sighted, skepticism from the scholarly, overinflation by the popular press, and panting expectation from potential patients. Only after a generation or so is their worth fully established.

The doubt and trouble that afflicted penicillin a generation ago have given way to universal praise and acceptance. Moreover, penicillin led the way for creation of a whole new family of medicines, many of which far outstrip their progenitor in power and range.

In all these aspects the future of interferon will likely be much the same. In their older years, today's young adults will almost certainly find interferon among the arsenal of common treatments their physician will have handy to help them. Some of these old folks will be given the opportunity to try new "biologicals," sophisticated hormone-like proteins being tested to supplant interferon as the sole cell modulating medication.

When the folks of this time feel colds coming on, they will get prescriptions for interferon nasal spray. It will be kept under prescription because doctors will want to make sure those most likely to suffer side effects avoid it.

When they are stricken by chronic or unusually severe virus infections, interferon will be used to hold the disease in check until a vaccine can be prepared or until the patient is better able to fight it off. In a few cases, interferon therapy strong enough to wipe out the infection will be used. Most often, doctors will want the patient to get a chance to develop antibodies to the disease, so it won't recur.

When people need transplanted organs, interferon will become a lifeline that wards off virus infections during the postoperative period and keeps the body from rejecting the transplanted organ. This may require treatment for days, weeks, or even a lifetime. Here the side effects don't matter much. Whatever they are, they will be less severe than rejection, reaction, and death.

And the treatment for cancer in these days will be much like the procedure for problems like a malfunctioning prostate or diabetes today. The disease won't be pleasant, not by any stretch of the imagination; it will still be traumatic and dangerous. But the treatment will reduce the fear in most cases from doom to discomfort and will offer effective therapy without deadly, permanent side effects.

A cancer patient might still be rushed into surgery or radiation for the removal of the initial tumor. Then, interferon therapy will begin. The protein will help prevent metastases, so cancer doesn't spread throughout the body. It will also help keep the patient strong and virus-infection-free so that any other needed treatments will have less sting.

A few patients may need to remain on interferon therapy the rest of their lives because they have high risk profiles, or because their cancer has a high incidence of fatal return. Here again, the side effects of interferon should be far preferable to the disease.

Interferon may also play some part in cancer prevention. When a group of people have been targeted as high risk potential cancer victims, they will undergo preventative interferon treatment in the hopes that the protein will keep cancer colonies from forming.

When will interferon emerge from the labs and clinics and land on doctors' shelves? Not fast enough to make very many people happy. But the development of a new drug takes time because no one—not in science, medicine, government, or business—wants to let a mistake invade the lives of millions of trusting patients. Patience and meticulous double-checking of attributes, side effects, dosages, methods of treatment, variable influences, and every other possible factor are necessary to make sure that the public is being presented with a safe, predictable treatment.

Today, researchers can say without hesitation that interferon works. What they need to be able to say before they can bring a drug to the market is: Interferon works here and doesn't work there. Interferon performs better here than it does there. Interferon given this way is better than interferon given that way. Interferon should never be given to this kind of person, it can always be safely given to that kind of person.

And, most important, interferon works this way *because* . . .

The protein must be studied and understood before it can be unleashed in the maze of situations that confront doctors in practice. This process takes years, and its course can be altered by unexpected blocks and twists. Given smooth sailing, however, interferon's course should follow a timetable like this:

1981. Genetically engineered interferon is produced, tested by governments, approved for clinical trials, and used in limited human trials. Synthetic interferon from sequencing may also appear. More detailed reports of the studies with natural interferon will come out.

1982. Results of genetically engineered interferon studies will begin to trickle out. The aggressive companies behind these tests will push for government approval to market as quickly as possible. If the tests look good, they'll get it. As soon as interferon is approved for marketing, supply limitations will vanish. The price will plummet as genetic engineering firms and pharmaceutical companies jockey for a share of the huge market.

1983. Drawing upon the huge supply of interferon, companies begin testing, and shortly thereafter marketing, interferon nasal sprays for limited use. It's still not exactly cheap, but a professional person could afford it for occasional use. Interferon becomes accepted as a treatment against rabies, eliminating the painful rabies shots that are now used.

1984. Genetic engineering companies begin announcing a second generation of biologicals growing out of their understanding of interferon. Some are more specific in action, some broader and milder. Some act only in certain parts of the body. Some are linked to enzymes that serve as triggers, so they don't snap into action until they hit a situation that strips away the enzyme-carrier.

1985. An aging scientist, in his memoirs, will look back and write: "Amazing as it may seem today, in the late 1970s and early 1980s there were many people, even many scientists, who doubted that interferon would ever have a role in medicine. If only they could be here now."

NOTES

Most of the information in this book came from oral interviews given by the experts noted in the text. To keep the notes manageable—since this is a book for a general audience—we have skipped repetitive references to interviews, and noted only the material drawn from published sources.

Introduction

1. A more detailed account of this embroglio can be found in "What Next for Interferon?" by Stephanie Yanchinski in *New Scientist*, September 25, 1980.
2. For the full statement of the problems between researchers and interferon recipients see "What Not to Say about Interferon," *Nature*, June 26, 1980.
3. Ibid.

Chapter 2

1. This quote is from testimony by Mathilde Krim before U.S. Representative Claude Pepper's Select Committee on Aging, June 19, 1979. A review of testimony by interferon experts can be found in *Cancer Letter*, June 29, 1979.
2. Quoted by Albert Rosenfeld, IF, *Life*, July, 1979.
3. Quoted on *NOVA*, a PBS television program produced by WGBH, Boston, and shown at various times on public television stations during 1980. The segment was titled: *The Big IF*.
4. Some of the information on Dr. Gutterman comes from an excellent profile that appeared in the Spectator column, *Houston City Magazine*, December 1980.
5. Krim's testimony at the Pepper hearings noted above.
6. Strander's testimony at the Pepper hearings.
7. The Sloan-Kettering letter can be found in the Science Times section of the *New York Times*, June 17, 1980.

Chapter 3

1. Merigan, Thomas, "Interferon as a Therapeutic Agent," *New England Journal of Medicine*, January 4, 1979.
2. Quoted by Kristin White, "Interferon: The Miracle Cure?", *Science and Living Tomorrow*, September 1980.
3. The standard technical work on how interferon works is: Stewart, W.E., *Interferons and Their Actions* (CRC Press, Chicago, 1977), a collection of reports by experts in various aspects of study in the field. This quote comes from Chapter 9: Krim, Mathilde and Saunders F. Kingsley, "Prophylaxis and Therapy with Interferons."

Chapter 4

1. The Epsteins' work is noted in two papers: "Genes Coding for Sensitivity to IF and Soluble Superoxide Dismutase are Linked in Mouse and Man . . ." *Proceedings of the National Academy of Science*, April 1980; "Assignment of the Genes for Sensitivity to Interferon . . . ," *Annals of the New York Academy of Sciences*, Volume 350, pp.171–173, 1980.
2. Keay, Susan and Grossberg, Sidney, "Interferon Inhibits the Conversion of 3T3-L1 Mouse Fibroblasts into Adipocytes," *Proceedings of the National Academy of Sciences*, July 1980.
3. See Chapter 3, number 3.

Chapter 5

1. Quoted by Kevin McKean in an Associated Press story on interferon recipients. It ran on April 27, 1980 in the *Staten Island Advance* under the headline "Is Interferon the 'Magic Bullet' that will Rip Holes in Cancer?" and in other papers at about the same time.
2. Mary Malone's story is related by Hal Lancaster in "Desperate Ones: Cancer Victims Plead to Receive Interferon, But Few Succeed," *Wall Street Journal*, May 21, 1980.
3. See Chapter 1, footnote 2.

Chapter 6

1. See Chapter 2, footnote 3.

Chapter 7

1. These quotes are from written responses by Dr. Gutterman to questions about interferon.

Chapter 8

1. The American Cancer Society press release about interferon funding was issued on August 30, 1978.
2. These comments are from Nicholas von Hoffman's column on the op-ed page of the *Washington Post*, November 29, 1980.
3. See Chapter 3, footnote 2.

Chapter 9

1. "The Miracles of Spliced Genes," *Newsweek*, March 17, 1980.
2. Quoted by James Wilkinson, "Engineering a Genetic Revolution," *New Scientist*, March 6, 1980.
3. Swanson is quoted in the article noted above.
4. Genentech official quoted by Debra Whitefield, "Gene Mixing: A New Field for Industry," *Los Angeles Times*, March 10, 1980.
5. Quoted by Jeff Wheelwright, "Boom In the Bio Business," *Life*, May 1980.
6. Andreopolis, Spyros, "Gene Cloning by Press Conference," *New England Journal of Medicine*, March 27, 1980.
7. Quoted by Nicholas Wade, "Cloning Gold Rush Turns Basic Biology Into Big Business," *Science*, May 16, 1980.
8. Memorandum from Steiner to Harvard staff.

Chapter 10

1. Dr. Chin prepared a report: "The Urgent Need for Larger Scale Production of Interferon from Human Leukocytes," for Sloan-Kettering's Interferon Lab. His story of interferon and penicillin comes from that report.

BIBLIOGRAPHY

The amount of material written about interferon has reached staggering proportions over the past few years. An attempt to include everything would overwhelm a non-professional reader, so I've included here only those articles I feel will be understandable and readily available to most people.

"Antibody Zeroes in on Interferon." *Science News*, June 21, 1980.

"At Only $100 Trillion a Gram, This 'Miracle' Has a Future." *Science Digest*, April 1980.

Bloom, Barry R. "Interferons and the Immune System." *Nature*, April 17, 1980.

Burke, Derek. "The Status of Interferon." *Scientific American*, April 1977.

"Can Interferons Cure Cancer"? *Lancet*, June 2, 1979.

Cantell, Kari. "Towards the Clinical Use of Interferon." *Chemtech*, September 1979.

"Engineered E. Coli Produce Interferon." *Nature*, January 24, 1980.

"Engineering a Genetic Revolution." *New Scientist*, March 6, 1980.

"Gene Mixing, a New Field for Industry." *Los Angeles Times*, March 10, 1980.

"Gene Transfer Given a New Twist." *Science*, April 25, 1980.

Hixson, Joseph. "Can Interferon Cure Cancer"? *New West*, January 15, 1979.

"How Interferon Interferes." *Scientific American*, May 1979.

"Immunology: Complexity Yielding to Research." *Chemical and Engineering News*, September 22, 1980.

"Industry of Life: Birth of the Gene Machine." *New York Times*, June 29, 1980.

"Interfering with Cancer." *Scientific American*, April 1979.

"Interferon." *Medical World News*, October 16, 1978.

"Interferon: Learning About How it Works." *Science*, June 22, 1979.

"Interferon: Medicine for Cancer and the Common Cold"? *Saturday Review*, November 25, 1978.

"Interferon: On the Threshold of Clinical Application. *Science*, June 15, 1979.

"Interferon Protects Kidney Transplants." *New Scientist*, July 12, 1979.

"Interferon: The Body's Own Wonder Drug." *Saturday Review*, October 13, 1979.

"Interferon: The Explosion Continues." *Science News*, November 22, 1980.

"Interferon, Virus Foe, Comes of Age." *New York Times*, December 26, 1980.

"Interferon was Considered for John Wayne." *Los Angeles Herald-Examiner*, June 14, 1979.

Isaacs, Alick. "Interferon." *Scientific American*, May 1961.

Journal of Interferon Research. A new professional journal devoted entirely to news of work in the interferon field. Of interest only to those who want extremely detailed information. Subscription: $45 from Mary Ann Liebert, Inc., 500 E. 85th St., New York, NY 10028.

Lancaster, Hal. "Cancer Victims Plead to Receive Interferon, But Very Few Succeed." *Wall Street Journal*, May 21, 1980.

Leff, David. "Interferon." *American Cancer Society Views*, Winter 1979.

Medical World News, July 7, 1980: several articles on interferon.

Medical World News, December 8, 1980: several articles on interferon.

"New Genetic Technologies: Prospects and Hazards." *Technology Review*, February 1980.

New York Times, June 17, 1980: numerous stories on Supreme Court genetic engineering decision; also includes the letter from Mathilde Krim and staff on interferon research.

Rosenfeld, Albert. "IF." *Life Magazine*, July 1979.

"Spliced Genes Get Down to Business." *Science News*, March 29, 1980.

"The Big IF in Cancer." *Time*, March 31, 1980.

"The Miracle of Spliced Genes." *Newsweek*, March 17, 1980.

"Viruses Lurking in Cells Suspected as Cause of a Host of Diseases." *New York Times*, December 23, 1980.

"What Not to Say About Interferon." *Nature*, June 26, 1980.

Wheelwright, Jeff. "Boom in the Bio Business." *Life Magazine*, May 1980.

White, Kristin. "Bacterial Interferon, Major New Source"? *Medical Tribune*, February 20, 1980.

________. "Interferon: The Promise and Reality." *Medical Tribune*, October 4, 1978.

Yanchinski, Stephanie. "What Next for Interferon"? *New Scientist*, September 25, 1980.

INTERFERON RESEARCH

Further research on interferon and interferon research can be obtained from a number of organizations and hospitals on both sides of the Atlantic. If you wish to know more about what is happening in the field, write to these sources for up-to-date information. Don't telephone them because they are extremely busy and can respond far better to letters, and don't ask them where you can get interferon. They can give out information, but they can't give out interferon, nor can they promise to get anyone onto an interferon testing program. Use these addresses for background information only. The chief sources of information in the United States are as follows:

American Cancer Society
777 Third Ave.
New York, NY 10017

American Committee of the Weizman Institute of Science
515 Park Ave.
New York, NY 10022

Interferon Evaluation Laboratory
Memorial Sloan-Kettering Cancer Center
1275 York Ave.
New York, NY 10021

The chief sources for information about interferon research in the United Kingdom are given below, though remember that these establishments can only provide you with information about interferon research. And, like their counterparts in the United States, they can only respond to letters:

Imperial Cancer Research Fund
Lincolns Inn Field
London

Department of Biological Sciences
University of Warwick
Coventry
Warwickshire CV4 7AL

Common Cold Unit
Coombe Road
Salisbury
Witlshire SP2 8BW

Division of Communicable Diseases
Clinical Research Centre
Watford Road
Harrow
Middlesex HA1 3UJ

Ludvig Institute for Cancer Research
The Medical School
Hills Road
Cambridge CB2 2QH

Wellcome Foundation
Langley Park
Beckenham
Kent

GLOSSARY

Anecdotal Study. A scientific study that draws conclusions from observation of an informal group of subjects, without the balance of a control group.

Antibody. A protein that reacts with a certain type of invasive material by linking with it and blocking its activity.

Chemotherapy. Treatment of cancer with drugs.

Chromosome. Thread-like strand of genetic material found in the nuclei of cells.

Cloning. Creation of an exact genetic replica of an organism.

Controlled study. A scientific test in which participants are split into two groups. The experimental group receives the material being tested and the control group does not. The differences in response of the two groups point up the material's actions.

DNA. A nucleic acid that is the basis for the storing of genetic messages on chromosomes.

Double-blind study. A controlled study in which neither the experimenters nor the subjects know who is receiving the treatment in question and who is receiving a placebo. Double-blind procedures eliminate the possibility of psychological clues passing from tester to subject that could affect responses.

E. coli. A microorganism found in the human colon that contains plasmids and is used frequently in genetic engineering.

Enzyme. Chemically active proteins that promote life processes without being changed or destroyed by them. Enzymes are the workhorses of our body chemistry.

Fibroblast interferon. Interferon derived from cells of the connective muscle tissues.

Gene. The basic unit of inheritance; a short length of chromosome that determines a specified biological action.

Genetic engineering. The process by which organisms can be induced to produce specified biological actions of chemicals by altering the composition of its genetic makeup.

Hepatitis. A viral inflammation of the liver, often chronic.

Herpes. A family of virus diseases characterized by open sores on the skin.

Hodgkin's disease. A cancer of the lymph nodes.

Hormone. A chemical messenger, produced by the endocrine gland. Hormones can cause reactions at remote parts of the body by travelling through the bloodstream.

Immune system. A complex range of bodily reactions that protect cells from intrusive elements. Its core is a group of different types of cells that identify unnatural influences in the body and attack them.

Interferoid. An interferon molecule that has been stripped of the sugars that are attached to each end of it.

Interferon. Any of a family of proteins produced by cells in the presence of viral infection (or conditions that ape viral infections) that induce in other cells protective measures against their own subjugation. Interferon consists of a long string of amino acids with sugar molecules on either end.

Leukocyte interferon. Interferon produced from human white blood cells. These cells are sometimes also known as buffy coats.

Lymphoblastoid interferon. Interferon derived from lymphatic system cells that have reverted to their undifferentiated state. Lymphoblastoid cells are often the result of lymph cancer.

Lymphocyte. A cell produced by the lymphatic system which is active in immune responses.

Killer Cell. An immune system cell that can recognize and attack an invader only after being triggered by an antibody.

Lymphoma. Cancer of the lymph tissue.

Macrophages. Large white blood cells that surround and dissolve invading cells in the blood.

Melanoma. Skin cancer characterized by dark pigments.

Metastasis. The spread of colonies of cancer cells from the site of the original outbreak to various parts of the body. The cells move through the blood, lymph, and other body systems.

Modality. A method of treatment.

Monoclonal antibody. An antibody that reacts with one molecule only. Most antibodies react with a family of similar chemicals, not just one.

Myeloma. Cancer of the bone marrow.

Namalva. A line of cells taken from a victim of Burkitt's lymphoma which have been kept alive in laboratories for use in experimentation.

Natural killer cells (NK Cells). A group of immune system cells that can recognize and attack invasive cells without first being triggered by an antibody.

Osteogenic sarcoma. A cancer that breaks out in the long bones of adolescents. Characterized by swift metastasis.

Papilloma. Benign but recurring throat tumors that can cause death by choking.

Placebo. A preparation with no medical effect that is given to experimental patients to test the power of their minds to generate healing. A placebo can also serve as a neutral medium for use on control groups.

Plasmid. A strand of DNA that is twisted into a ring. Genetic engineers can snip pieces of the ring and fuse into the gap new pieces of genetic information from other cells or organisms.

Protein. A long chemical chain made up of amino acids linked by peptides.

Recombinant DNA. Another name for genetic engineering. Refers to the plasmid that is broken and then recombined with new genetic material.

RNA. A nucleic acid that serves as the median for inheritance of DNA genetic messages during reproduction. It creates a mirror image of the DNA message that then serves as the basis for creation of a new DNA strand identical to the original.

M-RNA. Messenger RNA. A kind of RNA produced by the chromosomes for the purpose of instructing the cell to produce a specific chemical. The m-RNA carries the message of what the new chemical should be.

Species specificity. The limitation of a material's potency to the species from which it was derived.

Superinduction. A process for spurring the body to greater interferon levels by teasing it with a small dose of interferon, followed by a larger dose. The two-step approach induces the body to produce more interferon of its own than a single dose would.

Virus. An invader of cells that is made up of a protein sheath with a nucleic acid core. It is dependent upon living cells for life and reproduction.

INDEX

Index

Index